Exercise for Aging Adults

Gail M. Sullivan • Alice K. Pomidor

Editors

Exercise for Aging Adults

A Guide for Practitioners

Second Edition

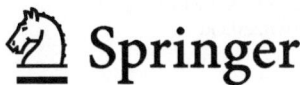 Springer

Editors
Gail M. Sullivan
UConn Center on Aging
University of Connecticut School of
Medicine
Farmington, CT, USA

Alice K. Pomidor
Florida State University (retired)
Tallahassee, FL, USA

ISBN 978-3-031-52927-6   ISBN 978-3-031-52928-3   (eBook)
https://doi.org/10.1007/978-3-031-52928-3

This Springer imprint is published by the registered company Springer Nature Switzerland AG
The registered company address is: Gewerbestrasse 11, 6330 Cham, Switzerland

Paper in this product is recyclable.

Introduction to the Second Edition

We continue to observe medications, herbals, foods, and now cannabidiol (CBD) products marketed as anti-aging products or cures for age-related problems—osteoarthritis, osteoporosis, urinary complaints, loss of strength—you name it. In earlier times, these products were referred to as "snake oil" and promoted by persons of dubious backgrounds. As geriatricians who base our recommendations on the best available evidence, this trend concerns us deeply. While commercial entities reap the profits, older adults around the world fail to benefit from one of the most effective and safest "medicines" found: exercise. This book is our way to encourage health professionals—usually highly trusted by older adults—to actively promote exercise during conversations with older individuals, regardless of setting, comorbid medical problems, or current function. All older adults need regular physical activity to maintain or improve function, treat many age-related medical conditions, and enhance their chances of successful aging. We know personally how hard it can be to integrate these exercise conversations, prescriptions, and physical activity programs into one's current practice. Yet it is incredibly gratifying when patients reclaim their independence, improve symptoms, or re-acquire a sense of vitality. For some older individuals, maintaining rather than improving function is the most realistic aim, and this goal is strongly preferred by older adults and their loved ones.

For this second edition, we added two chapters to address categories of older adults requiring counseling and encouragement to safely exercise: older athletes who want to exercise at high levels of frequency and/or intensity and older adults with pain due to common conditions such as osteoarthritis. Exercise is an effective single or adjunctive treatment for several painful conditions, yet not uniformly recommended. Older adults who seek to maintain or achieve a high level of performance—regardless of whether they choose to compete—need to adjust their regimens for success. Hence, Chaps. 11 and 12 are new chapters addressing these gaps.

We continue to be inspired by our patients. They provide portraits of successful aging in the face of inevitable age-related physical changes and new medical problems. Our patients help us to visualize and accept our own aging and our struggles to maintain exercise regimens. We are moved by the decision of a favorite patient to move 3000 miles to a new retirement community, closer to her family. Before she left her home of many decades, she lined up partners in her new locale for two hobbies of doubles tennis and creating math problems. She has enjoyed playing weekend tennis for many years; when one of us encouraged her to exercise more days of the week and include other exercise components, she took up senior karate. She is 90 years old and aging successfully despite a host of medical issues.

Another older adult who inspires us is a woman met while walking a steep path in the Scottish Highlands. She took up walking in her late 60s when her husband died, after a lifetime of being a self-described "couch potato." At 79 years young and 5 feet 1 inch tall in her boots, she and her friend, aged 74 years, led the rest of the group of mixed ages. She highlights that it is *never* too late to start moving.

To date, there is no comparable substitute for exercise: no pill, no procedure, no injection that works as well. Exercise IS medicine. Our culture and health professional training have not sufficiently prepared us for easily integrating activity prescriptions into our healthcare practices and programs. We hope this book or individual book chapters can aid our fellow practitioners in their quest to get older adults moving.

Thank you for your work with older adults,

Gail and Alice

Contents

List of Contributors

Lobna Ali Louisiana State University Health Sciences Center, New Orleans, LA, USA

Ashley L. Artese Department of Exercise Science and Health Promotion, Florida Atlantic University, Boca Raton, FL, USA

Department of Exercise Science and Health Promotion, Charles E. Schmidt College of Science, Florida Atlantic University, Boca Raton, FL, USA

Jenna M. Bartley UConn Center on Aging and Department of Immunology, School of Medicine, University of Connecticut, Farmington, CT, USA

Jennifer S. Brach University of Pittsburgh, Pittsburgh, PA, USA

Cynthia J. Brown Louisiana State University Health Sciences Center, New Orleans, LA, USA

Kenneth Brummel-Smith College of Medicine, Florida State University, Tallahassee, FL, USA

Andreia N. Cadar UConn Center on Aging and Department of Immunology, School of Medicine, University of Connecticut, Farmington, CT, USA

Tricia Creel MDT Education Solutions, Atlanta, MO, USA

Jacob Earp Department of Kinesiology, University of Connecticut, Storrs, CT, USA

Madeleine E. Hackney Department of Medicine, Emory University School Medicine, Atlanta VA Health Care System, Center for Visual and Neurocognitive Rehabilitation, Atlanta, GA, USA

Jason R. Jaggers Department of Health and Sport Sciences, University of Louisville, Louisville, KY, USA

Gardenia A. Juarez University of Pittsburgh, Pittsburgh, PA, USA

Kristi M. King Department of Health and Sport Sciences, University of Louisville, Louisville, KY, USA

Lynn B. Panton Florida State University, Tallahassee, FL, USA

Alice K. Pomidor Florida State University (retired), Tallahassee, FL, USA

Barbara Resnick Organizational Systems and Adult Health, School of Nursing, University of Maryland, Baltimore, MD, USA

Gail M. Sullivan UConn Center on Aging, University of Connecticut School of Medicine, Farmington, CT, USA

Joseph D. Vondrasek Cardiovascular and Applied Physiology Laboratory, Department of Health, Nutrition, and Food Sciences, Florida State University, Tallahassee, FL, USA

Joseph C. Watso Cardiovascular and Applied Physiology Laboratory, Department of Health, Nutrition, and Food Sciences, Florida State University, Tallahassee, FL, USA

Chapter 1
The Physiology of Aging and Exercise

Andreia N. Cadar and Jenna M. Bartley ⓘ

Key Points
- Biological aging, which drives age-related organ system dysfunctions, does not always align with chronological aging.
- Age-related alterations in nervous, musculoskeletal, and cardiovascular systems affect physical function to the greatest degree.
- Frailty is a multifactorial, multidimensional syndrome that is characterized by increased vulnerability to various stressors.
- Exercise targets multiple hallmarks of aging, as well as frailty, and can preserve many system-level declines related to aging.

Introduction

Aging is associated with the accumulation of molecular and cellular damage that leads to dysfunction and decline in many tissues and body systems [1]. Aging is a natural and universal process, yet interventions, such as exercise, can affect these changes in tissues and body systems. Older adults who complain about loss of strength, balance, and overall difficulties with activities of daily living may assume or be told, "it's just something that happens as you get older." The centuries long quest for the "fountain of youth," has not yielded a magic anti-aging pill to reverse the aging clock and rejuvenate older adults to their youthful function. Although no pill exists, decades of research show that exercise can improve age-related functional loss, while also reducing the risk of obesity, cardiovascular disease, cognitive

A. N. Cadar · J. M. Bartley (✉)
UConn Center on Aging and Department of Immunology, School of Medicine, University of Connecticut, Farmington, CT, USA
e-mail: jbartley@uchc.edu

© The Author(s), under exclusive license to Springer Nature Switzerland AG 2024
G. M. Sullivan, A. K. Pomidor (eds.), *Exercise for Aging Adults*,
https://doi.org/10.1007/978-3-031-52928-3_1

declines, and other age-related dysfunctions [2–5]. While the benefits of exercise are clear, they are often overlooked by clinicians and older adults alike. Fortunately, studies demonstrate that regular exercise, even when started late in life, can improve strength, endurance, balance, and overall quality of life in older adults.

This chapter describes the physiology of aging and its relationship to mobility and exercise interventions. Through a boom in aging research, common pathways, or hallmarks, of aging have been unveiled. In describing aging physiology, this chapter will discuss how exercise can target these hallmarks of aging and thus improve lifespan and healthspan in older adults.

Biology of Aging

First, it is crucial to differentiate *chronological* and *biological aging*. Chronological aging refers to the amount of time that has passed since one's birth, while biological aging refers to the level of dysfunction in cellular and molecular processes associated with aging. Although both are important to consider when addressing an individual's overall health, biological aging may be more indicative of robustness and resilience. For example, although two individuals share the same age, their ability to live independently, execute activities of daily living and maintain their hobbies and social roles may differ greatly.

Hallmarks of Aging

Aging research has identified many cellular and molecular hallmarks of aging [1, 6]. These hallmarks of aging manifest during normal aging, accelerate aging when experimentally aggravated, and retard the normal aging process when experimentally ameliorated. The currently identified hallmarks of aging are shown in the left boxes in Fig. 1.1 and several are discussed below. The cellular and molecular changes underlie the biological process of aging and are also interconnected in their physiological effects. These hallmarks are extensively reviewed elsewhere (see [1, 6]) and select hallmarks are expanded upon below. Understanding the different hallmarks allow us to understand how exercise benefits aging physiology.

Inflammation

Inflammation has been described as a double-edged sword. Although inflammation is essential for the immune response to infection and some aspects of regeneration, it can be detrimental at high levels or when dysregulated. When this occurs, inflammation may lead to cell death of healthy cells or organ failure. Age-related increases

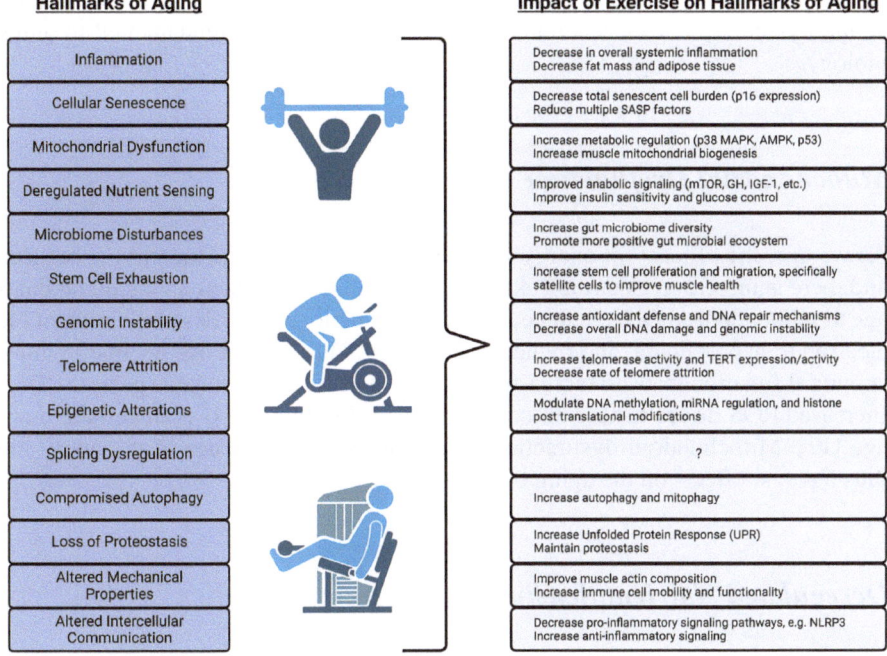

Fig. 1.1 The hallmarks of aging and impact of exercise. The hallmarks of aging are denoted on the left and the ways that exercise benefits these specific hallmarks are notated on the right. Figure created with BioRender.com

in basal, sterile inflammation, termed *inflammaging* [7], has become a major area of aging research as it effects nearly all other hallmarks of aging. Increased low-grade, chronic inflammation is associated with common complaints of older adults, such as body and joint pain, insomnia, and difficulty breathing. Excessive inflammation can lead to muscle catabolism, sarcopenia, and overall reduced function. *Frailty,* a clinical syndrome of older adults that indicates increased vulnerability to adverse health outcomes, is also characterized by excessive inflammation [8–10].

Cellular Senescence

Cellular senescence and inflammation are highly related hallmarks of aging. Cellular senescence refers to the irreversible proliferation arrest that occurs when cells experience cellular stressors, such as DNA damage or oxidative stress. Although senescent cells are primarily in an irreversible state of cell cycle arrest, they remain metabolically active and secrete a variety of pro-inflammatory cytokines, chemokines, and proteases [11]. In healthy young adults, these cells are readily cleared by the immune system. With aging, senescent cells accumulate in multiple tissues and are associated with age-related conditions, including frailty, osteoarthritis, and metabolic dysfunction. This accumulation of senescent cells is fundamental to aging biology.

Mitochondrial Dysfunction

As we age, the efficacy of energy generation through the mitochondria is reduced and there is increased electron leakage. This is due to many factors, including damage to mitochondrial DNA, reduced mitochondrial biogenesis, destabilization of the electron transport chain, and reduced mitophagy. This progressive decline in mitochondrial function leads to increased production of reactive oxygen species (ROS). Increased ROS drives further mitochondrial deterioration and overall cellular damage [12]. Mitochondrial dysfunction affects all cells and tissues of the body, and thus has vast effects on the aging body systems [1].

Deregulated Nutrient Sensing

There are many different nutrient sensing and signaling pathways throughout the body. With age, many of the nutrient sensing and signaling system pathways are dysregulated. For example, growth hormone (GH) and insulin-like growth factor 1 (IGF-1) pathways have been linked to longevity, through genetic mutations or interventions, in multiple species [13]. Indeed, the most well-known lifespan intervention, dietary restriction, targets these pathways to slow down cell growth and metabolism, which may be the mechanism to avoid cellular damage accumulation. Levels of GH, IGF-1, and other key anabolic hormones such as testosterone decline during aging. Hormone declines and dysregulation are accompanied by overall decreased anabolic molecular signaling and *anabolic resistance* with age. Anabolic resistance is the blunted muscle protein synthesis response to an anabolic signal, such as exercise or a protein dose [14, 15].

Microbiome Disturbances

Age-associated changes in the diversity, composition, and function of the gut microbiota occur with aging, but their effects are incompletely understood. Gut microbiome patterns are influenced by diet, medication, obesity, and physical activity, as well as age. There is increased intestinal permeability that is sometimes referred to as "leaky gut" [6]. In totality, these microbiome changes and leaky gut lead to a chronic low-grade systemic inflammation, which may contribute to overall inflammaging.

Stem Cell Exhaustion

Due to stem cell exhaustion, the regenerative potential of almost all tissues decreases with aging [16]. Hematopoietic stem cell exhaustion leads to impaired immune responses. Mesenchymal stem cell exhaustion leads to osteoporosis and other conditions. Satellite stem cells, specific to muscle, also are impaired and lead to sarcopenia. Overall, stem cell exhaustion with age reduces the regenerative potential of many different tissues and the accumulated cell damage cannot be repaired [1].

Other Hallmarks of Aging

With age, DNA damage accumulates particularly in telomeres. As DNA repair methods are insufficient with age, this leads to genomic instability and telomere attrition, two more hallmarks of aging [1, 6]. Epigenetic alterations, such as changes in acetylation and methylation of DNA and/or histones, also occur with aging and drive age-related transcriptional changes [17]. Dysregulated RNA splicing also occurs and leads to additional problems with gene transcription. With age, proteostasis loss occurs, in which unfolded proteins are not adequately refolded and there is inadequate degradation of these unfolded proteins [18]. Intercellular communication changes with age [1, 6]. Mechanical properties of cells also change which leads to overall reduced motility of many cell types, such as immune cells.

Aging of Body Systems

All major body systems—skeletal, muscular, nervous, endocrine, cardiovascular, lymphatic, respiratory, digestive, urinary, and reproductive—experience age-related declines (see Fig. 1.2). Of these, changes to the skeletal, muscular, nervous, cardiovascular, and respiratory systems have the largest effects on overall function.

Aging Skeletal System

Peak bone mass is normally achieved in the third decade of life. Over time there is a gradual reduction in bone mass, which is accelerated in women following menopause [19]. Decreases in bone mineral density (BMD), measured by dual X-ray absorptiometry (DXA), cause bones to become more fragile. When BMD falls one standard deviation below the average BMD for a healthy, young adult, bone is considered *osteopenic* [20]. When BMD is below 2.5 standard deviations from the average BMD for a healthy, young adult, bone is termed *osteoporotic* [20]. While it is estimated that heritable factors account for about 80% of our ability to achieve and

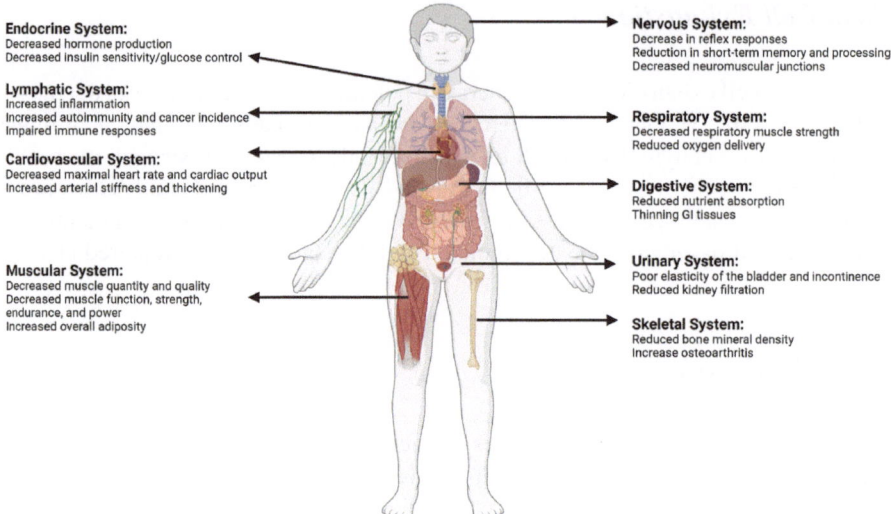

Endocrine System:
Decreased hormone production
Decreased insulin sensitivity/glucose control

Lymphatic System:
Increased inflammation
Increased autoimmunity and cancer incidence
Impaired immune responses

Cardiovascular System:
Decreased maximal heart rate and cardiac output
Increased arterial stiffness and thickening

Muscular System:
Decreased muscle quantity and quality
Decreased muscle function, strength, endurance, and power
Increased overall adiposity

Nervous System:
Decrease in reflex responses
Reduction in short-term memory and processing
Decreased neuromuscular junctions

Respiratory System:
Decreased respiratory muscle strength
Reduced oxygen delivery

Digestive System:
Reduced nutrient absorption
Thinning GI tissues

Urinary System:
Poor elasticity of the bladder and incontinence
Reduced kidney filtration

Skeletal System:
Reduced bone mineral density
Increase osteoarthritis

Fig. 1.2 The aging of the body systems. The body systems are heavily affected by aging with declines noted in each system. Figure created with BioRender.com

maintain BMD, modifiable factors, including exercise, contribute to bone health [21]. A sedentary lifestyle can accelerate bone loss and increase the risk for osteoporosis. Patients with osteoporosis have an increased risk for bone fractures from low trauma events, such as from a fall [20]. Hip fractures in osteoporotic adults can start a downward spiral of loss of independence, with an estimated only 25–33% of older adults regaining their pre-fracture level of function after recovery [22].

Aging Muscular System

Like bone, muscle mass declines begin by age 40 and accelerates in the 60s. With age there is a decrease in both muscle fiber number and muscle fiber size, with a preferential loss of type II fibers [23]. Type II fibers are fast twitch fibers and responsible for high force and fast contractions. This reduces the ability of older adults to generate maximal force quickly, like the motion necessary to "catch" oneself after a misstep, to prevent a fall. Deregulated nutrient sensing, anabolic resistance, inflammation, and satellite cell exhaustion all contribute to impaired muscle regeneration with age. Recent research has shown that satellite cells may also become senescent with age [24], which can further contribute to muscle decline through increased muscle-specific inflammation. Declines in muscle mass tend to be accompanied by increases in fat mass, both intramuscularly and overall, which can drive increased inflammation.

Sarcopenia is diagnosed based on muscle mass losses that are accompanied by muscle strength declines, decreased muscle quality, and overall reduced physical performance [25]. Sarcopenia prevalence ranges from 11 to 50% in individuals over the age of 80 and varies with underlying diseases and lifestyle differences. Multiple mechanisms drive sarcopenia, including reduced anabolic hormones, deregulated nutrient sensing, age-related neurodegeneration, and inflammatory cytokines [26]. Sedentary lifestyles are associated with sarcopenia and exercise programs are used to treat sarcopenia. Sarcopenia is associated with an increased risk of many adverse outcomes, such as falls, fractures, disability, hospitalization, and mortality [26].

Aging Nervous System

Both the central and peripheral nervous systems experience sharp declines with aging. Within the brain there is neuronal loss and decreased dendrite branches and interconnections. This is accompanied by reduced cerebral blood flow and impaired blood–brain barrier effectiveness. Neurotransmitters also are affected with aging. Overall, these changes lead to decreased capacity to send nerve impulses and slower information processing [27]. Processing response times generally increase, in memory, language, and reaction to auditory or visual stimuli. Peripherally, there is age-related neurodegeneration with loss of alpha motor neurons in the spinal cord, peripheral nerve fibers, and reduced neuromuscular junctions [28]. Since contractile characteristics of muscle are largely dictated by the motor nerves that innervate them, this aging change leads to motor unit loss and overall skeletal muscle fiber loss. Thus, the aging nervous system contributes to muscular decline, with prolonged reaction times and reduced proprioception.

Aging Cardiovascular System

The cardiovascular system, comprised of the heart muscle and vessels, transports nutrient-rich blood to and removes waste products from all cells of the body. Aging is associated with decreased cardiovascular capacity due to structural and other functional alterations. These changes produce a decrease in maximal oxygen uptake (VO_2 max) [29]. In older adults the aging heart shows myocardial hypertrophy and reduced left ventricular compliance, or relaxation [30]. The collagen content of cardiac tissue increases, particularly in the epicardial and endocardial layers of heart tissue, and the muscular myocardial layer becomes thicker and less compliant. As a result, the aging heart loses its capacity to increase stroke volume, the amount of blood ejected from the heart per beat, with increased exertion [30]. In addition, cardiac function is impaired by changes in the cardiac valves. Similar to the heart walls, the valves of the heart also thicken with calcium deposits and collagen.

Thickening impairs valve function, especially of the mitral and aortic valves. There is also an age-related reduction in maximal heart rate due to prolonged cardiac contraction and relaxation times with aging.

In circulatory vessels, arterial compliance decreases as the arterial walls thicken and calcify, which causes increased opposition to the flow of blood [30]. A reduction in vascular sensitivity to sympathetic nerve activity can impair vascular dilation. Reduced vessel diameter results in the heart having to work harder to push against greater resistance. Other vascular changes reduce renal, intestinal, skin, cerebral, and muscular perfusion. Blood flow is also impaired by diminished angiogenesis, which is the ability to grow new blood vessels. Plaque formation in the blood vessels, reduced elasticity of arteries, weakened venous valves, and fewer blood vessels together produce increased vessel resistance.

These cumulative aging cardiovascular system changes result in a reduced ability to elevate cardiac output, which affects exercise capacity and counseling around exercise adaptations, in older adults.

Aging Respiratory System

The respiratory system functions in conjunction with the cardiovascular system to determine functional capacity. The respiratory system delivers oxygen from the ambient air to the alveoli of the lungs where gases (oxygen and carbon dioxide) are exchanged. With aging, lung tissue loses elasticity, which reduces its ability to inflate and deflate [31]. As a result, in comparison to healthy younger adults, older adults have a lower vital capacity or ability to exchange large volumes of air. The reduction in vital capacity is largely due to an increased residual volume or volume of air remaining in the lungs after exhalation. Along with these structural changes of the lung, alveoli within the lung thicken, which reduces the surface area available for gas exchange between ambient air and capillary blood [31]. Together these changes lead to reduced oxygen exchange. Coupled with the cardiovascular declines of aging, functional capacity is reduced with potential symptoms of labored breathing and increased fatigue with exertion.

Aging of Other Body's Systems

While aging of the systems described above has the greatest effects on functional capacity of older adults, the endocrine, digestive, and lymphatic systems also impact function. Altered intercellular communication, deregulated nutrient sensing, and microbiota disturbances with aging affect the endocrine and digestive systems and contribute to reduced nutrient absorption and overall anabolic resistance. Impairment of the lymphatic system affects both innate and adaptive immunity, with dysfunctional responses from almost all immune cells. This leads to increased systemic inflammation with age, as well as impaired immune responses overall. Thus, older adults are at increased risk for infectious diseases, autoimmune disorders, and cancers, which can cause disability.

Frailty

Despite the universal hallmarks of cellular aging and resulting changes in body systems, there is a spectrum of aging. At any age some older adults are robust and resilient, while others are frail and non-resilient to stressors. The *frailty* syndrome is characterized by an increased vulnerability to physiological stressors and overall decreased physiological reserves and is associated with multiple poor health outcomes [8–10].

Frailty is defined through clinical factors and various measurement scales are in use. One frailty scale is based on clinical judgment and scores patients on a scale of 1 (very fit) to 8 (severe frailty), with a score of 9 reserved for those approaching the end of life [32]. While this scale appears straightforward, it is subjective and lacks ability to objectively classify older adults. The *Fried Frailty Phenotype* defines frailty as a clinical syndrome in which three or more of the following criteria are present: unintentional weight loss (10 lbs in past year), self-reported exhaustion, weakness (as measured by hand grip strength), slow walking speed, and a low level of physical activity. Individuals with a score of 0 are considered robust, 1–2 are considered pre-frail, and 3+ are considered frail [10]. *The Rockwood Frailty Index* is based on the concept that frailty is a consequence of interacting physical, psychological, and social factors; it may be considered a cumulative deficits model. The index is calculated from the number of deficits a patient has, divided by the number of deficits considered. A score of 0–0.1 is deemed non-frail, >0.1–0.21 is pre-frail, >0.21–0.45 is frail, and greater than 0.45 is most frail [33].

While different classifications of frailty result in varying prevalence of frailty, it is estimated that approximately 15% of community dwelling older adults (those 65 years and older) are frail. An additional 45% of community dwelling older adults are pre-frail [34]. Frailty is more common with advanced age and in women than men. There are also socioeconomic and racial disparities among frailty prevalence as well. While many factors contribute to frailty, chronic inflammation, hormonal changes, sarcopenia, and osteoporosis often underlie frailty diagnoses. Indeed, frailty is frequently associated with elevated inflammatory cytokines, mainly IL-6, and sarcopenia. Frail older adults are at an increased risk of mortality compared to non-frail older adults, with from 0.2 to 6-fold increased risk [35]. Furthermore, frail individuals are at greatly increased risk for disability. Thus, frailty represents an extreme maladaptive end of the aging spectrum, where older adults are highly vulnerable to health events due to their inability to effectively respond to stressors.

Exercise: The Anti-Aging Pill

Exercise and physical activity have extensive benefits, even when started later in life. While just a single session of exercise changes expression of almost ten thousand circulating molecular proteins and other signaling molecules, regular exercise has wide-ranging multifaceted benefits to multiple organ systems and improves longevity and health-span [2–4]. In fact, many aspects of age-related physiological declines mirror declines seen with disuse and deconditioning.

Regular exercise has beneficial effects on all major body systems. Regular exercise improves cardiovascular and respiratory function with increased cardiac output, VO_2 max, blood vessel health, and an overall decrease in risk factors for cardiovascular disease [36, 37]. Regular exercise prevents muscle loss with age and improves overall muscle quality, while also improving balance and motor coordination [38–40]. While aerobic endurance training improves peak oxygen consumption and muscle mitochondrial bioenergetics, resistance training increases muscle strength and mass. Further, exercise decreases systemic inflammation and increases anabolic signaling and protein synthesis, to prevent and reduce sarcopenia [40–43]. Exercise improves overall body composition and reduces adiposity in favor of muscle, which further benefits the hormonal and cytokine milieu by reducing adipose-derived pro-inflammatory signals and metabolic dysregulation [43]. Along with anabolic hormonal signaling, exercise decreases insulin resistance and improves gluconeogenesis and fatty acid metabolism [2, 4]. Osteoporosis risks are reduced by the effects of resistance exercise on bone metabolism [44]. Regular exercise improves hematopoietic stem cell function, immune responses to vaccination and infection, and lymphatic function [2–4, 45, 46].

These body system effects from exercise are driven by benefits at the molecular level (Fig. 1.1). While acute exercise causes a temporary increase in some inflammatory cytokines, regularly exercising reduces systemic inflammation. This is mediated through many mechanisms, including reduced overall adiposity, improved intercellular communication, and reduced total senescent cell burden [2–4]. Exercise downregulates pro-inflammatory pathways and allows for better intercellular communication. Exercise training can reduce markers of cellular senescence and components of the pro-inflammatory milieu from senescent cells in both adipose and muscle tissue [43, 47]. It also improves overall mitochondrial health and function. Research has shown that exercise can not only increase total mitochondria within skeletal muscle, but also improve mitochondrial function overall, evident through improved morphology and oxidative capacity [48]. Exercise increases telomerase activity and prevents overall telomere attrition with age. Exercise also increases DNA repair mechanisms and reduces unfavorable epigenetic alterations. Stem cell exhaustion is improved with exercise, with benefits evident within skeletal muscle satellite cells as well as hematopoietic stem cells. Thus, exercise improves the overall regenerative potential of multiple tissues with aging [2–4].

Furthermore, exercise increases autophagy and mitophagy and improves unfolded protein responses with better maintenance of proteostasis [49]. Deregulated nutrient sensing with aging is improved by exercise training. Signaling pathway improvements for multiple hormones are seen with exercise [2–4]. These improvements allow exercising older adults to overcome the general anabolic resistance seen with aging. Exercise can improve actin composition within muscle, as well as improve overall immune cell mobility and function.

Thus, exercise targets nearly all of the hallmarks of aging (Fig. 1.1, right side) with comprehensive benefits to multiple physiological systems. Importantly, these benefits are seen even when exercise is started later in life. Even in frail older adults, exercise demonstrates benefits in multiple dimensions.

Conclusions

Aging is associated with the accumulation of extensive molecular and cellular damage that leads to physiological declines in multiple body systems. While the "fountain of youth" has yet to be found, exercise targets multiple aspects of age-related declines, both at molecular and body system levels. Despite the strong evidence, only an estimated 26% of older adults engage in the recommended amount of regular physical activity [50]. A multicomponent exercise program that includes both aerobic and resistance training is essential to address physiologic declines typically seen with aging, to prolong health-span and promote healthy aging. Subsequent chapters of this book will address how to support more older adults to benefit from the magic, anti-aging, exercise pill.

References

1. Lopez-Otin C, et al. The hallmarks of aging. Cell. 2013;153(6):1194–217.
2. Carapeto PV, Aguayo-Mazzucato C. Effects of exercise on cellular and tissue aging. Aging. 2021;13(10):14522–43.
3. Goh J, et al. Targeting the molecular & cellular pillars of human aging with exercise. FEBS J. 2021;290(3):649–68.
4. Garatachea N, et al. Exercise attenuates the major hallmarks of aging. Rejuvenation Res. 2015;18(1):57–89.
5. Garatachea N, et al. Physical exercise as an effective antiaging intervention. Biomed Res Int. 2017;2017:7317609.
6. Schmauck-Medina T, et al. New hallmarks of ageing: a 2022 Copenhagen ageing meeting summary. Aging. 2022;14(16):6829–39.
7. Franceschi C, Campisi J. Chronic inflammation (inflammaging) and its potential contribution to age-associated diseases. J Gerontol A Biol Sci Med Sci. 2014;69(1):4–9.
8. Wilson D, et al. Frailty and sarcopenia: the potential role of an aged immune system. Ageing Res Rev. 2017;36:1–10.
9. Bandeen-Roche K, et al. Frailty in older adults: a nationally representative profile in the United States. J Gerontol A Biol Sci Med Sci. 2015;70(11):1427–34.
10. Fried LP, et al. Frailty in older adults: evidence for a phenotype. J Gerontol A Biol Sci Med Sci. 2001;56(3):M146–56.

11. Di Micco R, et al. Cellular senescence in ageing: from mechanisms to therapeutic opportunities. Nat Rev Mol Cell Biol. 2021;22(2):75–95.
12. Hekimi S, Lapointe J, Wen Y. Taking a "good" look at free radicals in the aging process. Trends Cell Biol. 2011;21(10):569–76.
13. Barzilai N, et al. The critical role of metabolic pathways in aging. Diabetes. 2012;61(6):1315–22.
14. Haran PH, Rivas DA, Fielding RA. Role and potential mechanisms of anabolic resistance in sarcopenia. J Cachexia Sarcopenia Muscle. 2012;3(3):157–62.
15. Rennie MJ. Anabolic resistance: the effects of aging, sexual dimorphism, and immobilization on human muscle protein turnover. Appl Physiol Nutr Metab. 2009;34(3):377–81.
16. Sharpless NE, DePinho RA. How stem cells age and why this makes us grow old. Nat Rev Mol Cell Biol. 2007;8(9):703–13.
17. Sierra MI, Fernandez AF, Fraga MF. Epigenetics of aging. Curr Genomics. 2015;16(6):435–40.
18. Koga H, Kaushik S, Cuervo AM. Protein homeostasis and aging: the importance of exquisite quality control. Ageing Res Rev. 2011;10(2):205–15.
19. Demontiero O, Vidal C, Duque G. Aging and bone loss: new insights for the clinician. Ther Adv Musculoskelet Dis. 2012;4(2):61–76.
20. Varacallo M, et al. Osteopenia. In: StatPearls. Treasure Island: StatPearls; 2022.
21. Morris JA, et al. An atlas of genetic influences on osteoporosis in humans and mice. Nat Genet. 2019;51(2):258–66.
22. Magaziner J, et al. Predictors of functional recovery one year following hospital discharge for hip fracture: a prospective study. J Gerontol. 1990;45(3):101–7.
23. Wilkinson DJ, Piasecki M, Atherton PJ. The age-related loss of skeletal muscle mass and function: measurement and physiology of muscle fibre atrophy and muscle fibre loss in humans. Ageing Res Rev. 2018;47:123–32.
24. Brack AS, Munoz-Canoves P. The ins and outs of muscle stem cell aging. Skelet Muscle. 2016;6:1.
25. Ardeljan AD, Hurezeanu R. Sarcopenia. In: StatPearls. Treasure Island: StatPearls; 2022.
26. Cruz-Jentoft AJ, et al. Sarcopenia: revised European consensus on definition and diagnosis. Age Ageing. 2019;48(4):601.
27. Lee J, Kim HJ. Normal aging induces changes in the brain and neurodegeneration progress: review of the structural, biochemical, metabolic, cellular, and molecular changes. Front Aging Neurosci. 2022;14:931536.
28. Hunter SK, Pereira HM, Keenan KG. The aging neuromuscular system and motor performance. J Appl Physiol. 2016;121(4):982–95.
29. Betik AC, Hepple RT. Determinants of VO2 max decline with aging: an integrated perspective. Appl Physiol Nutr Metab. 2008;33(1):130–40.
30. Ferrari AU, Radaelli A, Centola M. Invited review: aging and the cardiovascular system. J Appl Physiol. 2003;95(6):2591–7.
31. Schneider JL, et al. The aging lung: physiology, disease, and immunity. Cell. 2021;184(8):1990–2019.
32. Rockwood K, Theou O. Using the clinical frailty scale in allocating scarce health care resources. Can Geriatr J. 2020;23(3):210–5.
33. Searle SD, et al. A standard procedure for creating a frailty index. BMC Geriatr. 2008;8:24.
34. Ofori-Asenso R, et al. Global incidence of frailty and prefrailty among community-dwelling older adults: a systematic review and meta-analysis. JAMA Netw Open. 2019;2(8):e198398.
35. Ofori-Asenso R, et al. Frailty confers high mortality risk across different populations: evidence from an overview of systematic reviews and meta-analyses. Geriatrics. 2020;5(1):17.
36. El Assar M, et al. Effect of physical activity/exercise on oxidative stress and inflammation in muscle and vascular aging. Int J Mol Sci. 2022;23(15):8713.
37. Heckman GA, McKelvie RS. Cardiovascular aging and exercise in healthy older adults. Clin J Sport Med. 2008;18(6):479–85.
38. Cartee GD, et al. Exercise promotes healthy aging of skeletal muscle. Cell Metab. 2016;23(6):1034–47.

39. Rebelo-Marques A, et al. Aging hallmarks: the benefits of physical exercise. Front Endocrinol. 2018;9:258.
40. Rogeri PS, et al. Strategies to prevent sarcopenia in the aging process: role of protein intake and exercise. Nutrients. 2021;14(1):52.
41. Deutz NE, et al. Protein intake and exercise for optimal muscle function with aging: recommendations from the ESPEN Expert Group. Clin Nutr. 2014;33(6):929–36.
42. Griffen C, et al. Effects of resistance exercise and whey protein supplementation on skeletal muscle strength, mass, physical function, and hormonal and inflammatory biomarkers in healthy active older men: a randomised, double-blind, placebo-controlled trial. Exp Gerontol. 2022;158:111651.
43. Woods JA, et al. Exercise, inflammation and aging. Aging Dis. 2012;3(1):130–40.
44. Pinheiro MB, et al. Evidence on physical activity and osteoporosis prevention for people aged 65+ years: a systematic review to inform the WHO guidelines on physical activity and sedentary behaviour. Int J Behav Nutr Phys Act. 2020;17(1):150.
45. Domaszewska K, et al. Protective effects of exercise become especially important for the aging immune system in the Covid-19 era. Aging Dis. 2022;13(1):129–43.
46. Simpson RJ, et al. Exercise and the aging immune system. Ageing Res Rev. 2012;11(3):404–20.
47. Schafer MJ, et al. Exercise prevents diet-induced cellular senescence in adipose tissue. Diabetes. 2016;65(6):1606–15.
48. Zhang Y, Oliveira AN, Hood DA. The intersection of exercise and aging on mitochondrial protein quality control. Exp Gerontol. 2020;131:110824.
49. Escobar KA, et al. Autophagy and aging: maintaining the proteome through exercise and caloric restriction. Aging Cell. 2019;18(1):e12876.
50. Kruger J, Carlson SA, Buchner D. How active are older Americans? Prev Chronic Dis. 2007;4(3):A53.

Chapter 2
Benefits of Exercise for Older Adults

Gail M. Sullivan

Key Points
- Older adults benefit greatly from physical activity during daily routines and exercise, to prevent and treat chronic diseases and conditions commonly experienced in late life
- Exercise reduces hospitalizations, and improves function, mobility, and quality of life in older persons
- Exercise is generally well-tolerated in older adults, even in those at advanced age or with frailty
- Health care professionals as well as many older adults are unaware of the extensive benefits of exercise—the "miracle drug"—for older adults

Case: Part 1

Mr. and Mrs. Sampson are 80 years old. Mrs. Sampson has osteoporosis and osteoarthritis, with a past history of depression, and feels she has "slowed down." She becomes tired doing her housework. Her doctor told her, "It's your age, consider hiring a cleaner." She also worries about getting dementia, as her mother developed this in late life.

Mr. Samson had a small heart attack in the past and recently fell while walking outside on the lawn: he lost his balance. He feels he is getting weaker each year. His doctor told him he is "pre-diabetic" which was scary, as he gained only 25 pounds over the past few years.

They recently saw an advertisement for an expensive diet supplement that reverses aging and asked their daughter to order it. Their daughter, a community recreation director, responds that there *is* a wonder drug for aging and diseases: it's called EXERCISE. They are amazed and want to hear more.

G. M. Sullivan (✉)
UConn Center on Aging, University of Connecticut School of Medicine, Farmington, CT, USA
e-mail: gsullivan@uchc.edu

© The Author(s), under exclusive license to Springer Nature Switzerland AG 2024
G. M. Sullivan, A. K. Pomidor (eds.), *Exercise for Aging Adults*, https://doi.org/10.1007/978-3-031-52928-3_2

Introduction

Decades of research have shown that exercise delivers major benefits for maintaining independence and aging more successfully [1]. Many health professionals and older adults are aware that exercise is generally good for you, but less knowledgeable regarding the surprising array of benefits from daily physical activity and exercise training. Many conditions and diseases commonly occurring in older adults can be prevented, ameliorated, or treated with exercise. Changes that are often assumed to be due to aging, such as slow gait, unsteady balance, weight gain, joint pains, low energy, and slower reaction times, appear more a "dis-use" phenomenon, rather than inevitable with aging, and are avoided or improve with exercise. For some conditions, exercise is not only a primary but safer treatment, in comparison with pharmacologic choices [2]. The "Exercise is Medicine" movement expresses the need to consider exercise as a modality comparable to medicine for many health problems [3, 4]. On the cellular level, aging reverses or prevents many declines associated with aging (see Chap. 1). Thus, many experts view exercise as an "anti-aging pill."

Older adults and health professionals are also less cognizant that exercise can be safe for older adults including those with frailty syndrome. In fact, lack of exercise is more dangerous than exercise for most individuals; thus, many experts consider being sedentary a lethal condition [2]. Because of the demonstrated benefits from exercising, national and international groups have developed evidence-based exercise recommendations and promotion campaigns for *all* older adults [5–8]. Here, physical activity is defined as all physical activities that expend energy, whether in daily living, such as cooking, cleaning, and shopping, or specific exercises or sports. Exercise is a specific type of physical activity that is structured, planned, and carried out within a specific time period. Exercise includes movements for balance, muscle strength and power, endurance or aerobic capacity, and flexibility.

In short, most experts now consider increased physical activity and exercise to be not only hallmarks of, but also successful ingredients for successful aging [1] (see Tables 2.1 and 2.2).

Function and Mortality

For most older adults, maintaining independent function is a primary goal. In some individuals, loss of independence and becoming a burden on others are outcomes that are feared more than death. Longitudinal studies show that older adults lose physical functions—the ability to walk upstairs, balance while reaching for an object, or get out of a chair—over time, and this can be prevented by exercises, especially those for strength and balance [9, 10]. Preserving function as people age reduces disability and the resulting need for caregiver assistance in activities of daily living (ADL) [10]. Exercising three times a week or mobility training have

Table 2.1 Health benefits from exercise in older adults

Reduced risk of	Improved
All-cause mortality	Quality of life
Falls and fall-related injuries	Function
Cardiovascular mortality	Bone health
Cardiovascular disease	Pain relief, e.g., osteoarthritis
Stroke	Weight control
Hypertension	Sleep
Diabetes mellitus type 2	Possibly, cognition
Cancers, many	
Dementia	
Depression	
Anxiety	
Frailty	

Table 2.2 Exercise benefits for older adults with chronic health conditions

Condition	Benefits
Osteoarthritis	Decreased pain Improved physical function
Hypertension	Reduced cardiovascular disease progression and mortality
Diabetes mellitus type 2	Reduced cardiovascular mortality Improved hemoglobin A1C, blood pressure, body mass index, lipids
Hyperlipidemia	Improved lipid profile
Chronic obstructive pulmonary disease	Improved quality of life Improved dyspnea, fatigue, emotional control Improved hospitalizations Improved exercise capacity
Dementia	Improved function
Depression	Remission of symptoms Lower relapse rate
Cancer	Improved quality of life Improved fitness Reduced cancer mortality from breast, colorectal, prostate cancers Reduced all-cause mortality from breast, colorectal cancers
Frailty	Improved mobility, function, cognition

been shown to maintain and improve function in older adults, including individuals in long-term care facilities, who have chronic diseases, or who are frail [11–13]. A 2017 systematic review found that interventions with moderate physical activity levels and high memory, attention, coordination, balance, and social interactions were associated with larger benefits in ADL performance [14]. In contrast, a sedentary lifestyle is associated with reduced ability to perform ADLs and maintain independent function in older adults [5].

Lack of activity and exercise is highly associated with increased mortality in many observational studies, but whether this is an independent association is not clear [15, 16]. Is the association due to exercise effects on diseases (e.g., cardiovascular) and geriatric conditions (e.g., falls, fractures) or a direct effect of exercise on lifespan? Randomized controlled trials of exercise that account for all other variables affecting mortality have not been and likely will not be undertaken, given the known powerful effects of exercise on diseases and conditions that do shorten lifespan. A prospective cohort study using the US National Interview Survey, of half a million adults followed over 10 years, found that moderate level aerobic, vigorous level aerobic, and muscle-strengthening exercises were all associated with reduced all-cause, cardiovascular, and cancer mortality [17]. These mortality reductions were substantial: 50% lower for all-cause and cancer, and threefold reduction in cardiovascular mortality [17].

Exercise Benefits for Diseases and Conditions

Falls

Falls rise with age and increase the risk of serious injuries and fear of falling. More than one in four US adults aged 65 years or older falls each year [18]. The most consequential fall outcomes are fractures and head injuries, with associated high morbidity, functional decline, pain, and health care expenses. Many studies have shown that exercise, particularly balance activities, reduces falls in older adults with different physical abilities, medical conditions, and living settings. A Cochrane Collaboration review of community-dwelling older adults found a 23% reduction in falls and a 15% reduction in having more than one fall, with exercise [19]. Exercise interventions also reduced fall-related fractures and falls requiring medical attention, but the evidence for these outcomes was less certain due to lower numbers of studies and participants. Adverse effects were uncommon and primarily minor musculoskeletal complaints [19]. As a result, many organizations promote physical performance assessment and exercise for all older adults in their fall risk reduction guidelines [20].

Osteoporosis

Based on many observational studies and intervention trials, exercise is important for bone health [21]. Both older women and men suffer from osteopenia and osteoporosis, with decreases in bone mineral density and associated increased fracture risk. When combined with a high fall risk, this is a potent recipe for adverse outcomes. The fracture risk in men is less well recognized by health professionals and older individuals; in fact, the fracture rate is rising faster in men than in women, although both are increasing [3]. Regardless of site, fractures have a major impact on older adults and many do not recover their pre-fracture function despite complete bone healing. Immobilization and being sedentary accelerate bone loss, whereas weight-bearing and resistance (strengthening) exercises appear to maintain bone, in addition to beneficial effects on fall risk [3, 22]. Higher "doses" of exercise appear more beneficial [3, 22].

Many health professionals are cautious about suggesting strengthening exercises to older adults who have osteoporosis, for fear of causing harm, such as a fracture. But the evidence from studies does not support these fears, even with moderate to high-intensity exercise programs [21]. Rather than avoiding physical activity and exercise, experts recommend that older persons who have spinal fractures or multiple low-trauma fractures due to osteoporosis should limit impact beyond that of walking and/or start a program under supervision [21]. Experts also advise that those with spinal fractures should avoid extreme spinal flexion postures [21].

Osteoarthritis

Persons with osteoarthritis (OA), also known as degenerative joint disease, exhibit loss of articular cartilage with characteristic radiologic findings. OA is highly prevalent in older adults: virtually all older adults show evidence of osteoarthritis in at least one joint [3]. Prior joint trauma is associated with OA, but in most older adults OA is related to aging. Joint pain and stiffness are hallmarks and may lead individuals to avoid exercise and many daily activities; however, exercise is an effective treatment for both pain and stiffness (see Chap. 12). Evidence strongly supports exercise for knee and hip OA pain, in which endurance (aerobic) and resistance (strengthening) exercises are beneficial and comparable to steroid joint injections in efficacy. Stretching (flexibility) exercises also can improve stiffness and relieve pain. Studies also strongly support the role of exercise in managing back pain, highly prevalent in older adults, as well (see Chap. 12).

Many different exercise interventions have shown benefits for function and pain, thus, patient preference, other medical conditions, and access may guide exercise recommendations. Non-weight-bearing activities, such as pool-based or seated, are often suggested for individuals with OA who experience pain with standing or walking.

Experts recommend a more cautious approach to activities when joints appear actively inflamed, i.e., with fluid, heat, or redness of the joint, or when an exercise intervention increases pain. Stopping exercise entirely is not recommended, but rather stepping back to a lower level, changing to a different type of exercise (e.g., from resistance to endurance), or pausing and resuming when symptoms improve is suggested [3].

Hypertension, Cardiovascular, Cerebrovascular, and Peripheral Vascular Conditions

With increasing age, older adults are at high risk for vascular diseases. For many years health professionals and their patients believed that exercise would precipitate vascular events; many still do. While sudden vigorous exercise in previously sedentary individuals has been associated with adverse outcomes such as myocardial infarction, particularly in middle aged men, other types of exercise have not been [23]. Research strongly supports exercise for prevention and treatment of vascular conditions: hypertension, coronary vascular disease, cerebrovascular disease, and peripheral vascular disease [24].

Exercise is a well-accepted aspect of rehabilitation after cardiac events including myocardial infarction, angina pectoris, congestive heart failure, coronary bypass grafts, or percutaneous stents, with reductions in cardiac mortality, cardiac events, and hospitalizations, and improved quality of life [25]. Unfortunately, older adults are less likely to be referred for cardiac rehabilitation programs than other adults [26]. Recommendations for exercise in the setting of cardiovascular disease include first assessing exercise capacity and then an individualized program of endurance and resistance components. Persons with unstable angina, rest dyspnea, or recent (within a week) of myocardial infarct or stenting should delay the program until deemed stable. Coronary artery bypass patients should delay initiation longer, 4–6 weeks, pending surgeon approval [25].

Similarly, adults with stable congestive heart failure benefit from exercise, in quality of life, function, and congestive heart failure-related hospitalizations [25]. Exercise should be tailored to starting exercise capacity and most studies have used endurance (aerobic) exercises.

Cerebrovascular disease increases with age and strokes are greatly feared by older adults. Physical inactivity is a risk factor for hypertension, atherosclerosis, and diabetes mellitus, which are in turn strongly associated with cerebrovascular disease [3]. Thus, the benefit of exercise in reducing strokes may be through effects on these factors. In addition, many studies show the benefits of individualized exercise programs, for patients post-stroke, on function, walking speed, and quality of life. Some studies show benefits greater for exercise than for anti-coagulant and anti-platelet medications, for patients without known embolic risks [3].

Hypertension, particularly systolic hypertension, is increasingly common as adults age and increases the risk for cardio-, cerebro-, peripheral, and renovascular diseases, heart failure, and death [3]. Exercise is a first-line and adjunctive treatment for hypertension at any age, with fewer side effects in comparison with medications [2]. Both endurance—such as walking—and strength training programs have been well-studied [3]. Past research focused primarily on aerobic exercise, such as walking, for hypertension. A 2023 large meta-analysis, all age groups, found favorable results with many types of exercise for lowering systolic blood pressure: isometric exercise training (e.g., planks), combined training, dynamic resistance training, aerobic exercise, and high-intensity interval training [27].

Exercise has not been associated with causing strokes in older adults with hypertension, but experts recommend that extremely high blood pressures be controlled before increasing physical exertions [3]. The American College of Sports Medicine also advises against high-intensity dynamic or strength training with heavy weights, in persons with hypertension or heart failure [3].

For older adults with claudication—pain in the lower limbs—due to peripheral artery disease, exercise is a primary treatment, along with management of factors that promote vascular disease (smoking, Diabetes mellitus type 2 (DM2), hypertension, and hyperlipidemia). Unfortunately, pain may encourage older adults to stop exercising, which results in reduced fitness and facilitates disease progression. Multiple studies confirm the important benefits of various exercise modes in increasing walking distance, pain-free walking, and quality of life [28].

Diabetes and Lipids

DM2 also increases with age and is another condition that creates apprehension in older adults. DM2 is highly associated with vascular diseases, including myocardial infarction, stroke, peripheral vascular disease, renovascular disease, visual loss, and dementia, due to effects on large and small blood vessels. Exercise plays a role in preventing as well as managing DM2 [3]. Exercise can help with weight control, which is a risk factor for DM2. But exercise also independently lowers the risk of developing DM2. Exercise—whether endurance, strength, or a combination of both—is considered a cornerstone of DM2 treatment, and improves hemoglobin A1C level, insulin sensitivity, and fitness. Counseling regarding increasing physical activity should take into consideration an older adult's other health conditions, with additional discussions around avoiding hypoglycemia, especially for patients taking DM2 medications such as sulphonylureas, postprandial regulators, or insulin [3].

Hyperlipidemias—elevated cholesterol and triglycerides—confer additional risk for vascular diseases through increasing atherosclerosis. Many studies demonstrate the beneficial effects of exercise, both aerobic and resistance modalities, on lipids, and these effects are independent of weight loss. More improvements are seen if the duration or intensity of training is high. The improvements may be sufficient to avoid medications in some individuals with vascular event risks [3].

Chronic Obstructive Pulmonary Disease

Older adults with chronic obstructive disease (COPD) will experience over time increasing difficulty with physical activities and ADLs. In response, individuals may progressively reduce activities, which causes further reductions in strength and exercise capacity, and increases dyspnea (i.e., breathlessness). Pulmonary rehabilitation, a generally outpatient program over an average of 12 weeks, is designed to reverse this vicious cycle and specifically targets the underlying physiology, functional loss, and anxiety that occur in COPD, through exercise, education, and psychological support. Older persons with COPD often report that participation in such a program is a "game changer" in their lives. Unfortunately, pulmonary rehabilitation programs are not available in every area and may not be covered by insurance.

Strong evidence supports meaningful improvements in quality of life, dyspnea, fatigue, emotional control, hospitalizations, and exercise capacity from these programs [29]. Data suggests that the exercise component—which includes endurance and/or resistance exercises—of these programs has the greatest beneficial effect on outcomes [29]. Tailoring the program to a patient's other medical conditions as well as maintaining the oxygen saturation at 90% or higher is advised [3].

Mental Health

Depression, occurring alone or in association with conditions commonly experienced by older adults, such as stroke, can be managed with non-pharmacological approaches in some cases. Older adults often prefer treatment with non-medication strategies, such as talk therapy or exercise [30]. These approaches come with the advantage of fewer side effects than anti-depressant medications, which increase risks for falls and confusion in older adults. Exercise may also play a preventive role; epidemiologic studies show an inverse relationship between fitness and depression, and exercise and depression [3].

Studies find few treatment differences between exercise vs. medication treatment, and exercise vs. psychological therapy in treating depression, but confidence in the results is lessoned related to variable methods and potential bias [31]. Even in more severe depression, exercise may be as successful as medication treatment, but with slower effect [3]. Some studies suggest that relapse may be less frequent with exercise, but the exercise must be continued. Evidence for exercise stems primarily from aerobic, resistance, or mixed training interventions.

Anxiety is also commonly experienced by older adults, whether new or as a continuation of lifelong symptoms. Epidemiologic studies show that exercising is associated with less anxiety, but whether interventions can reduce anxiety is less certain. In randomized controlled trials, not focused on older adults, exercise reduced anxiety and stress-related symptoms. Studies of adults with anxiety related to disease conditions, such as COPD or cardiovascular disease, show reduced anxiety symptoms with exercise [3]. Aerobic exercise is the most studied type in these trials.

Sleep

About half of all older adults note problems sleeping, which are related to medical conditions (urinary frequency, joint pain, breathing problems), more fragmented sleep with age, and medications [32]. Non-pharmacological approaches are more attractive than sleep hypnotic drugs, which increase risks for falls and confusion in older persons. Exercise is effective in improving perceptions and objective measures of sleep quality in adults, but there are fewer studies in older adults [33]. Both moderate intensity aerobic exercise, such as walking or cycling, and mind-body exercise, such as yoga, have been effective over relatively short intervention periods, e.g., 2 months, in adults of mixed ages [33].

A 2020 systematic review of randomized controlled trials in *healthy* older adults concluded that exercise was highly effective in improving sleep measures, particularly interventions of moderate intensity, three times weekly, and continued over 12 weeks or more. Both combination programs and single exercise types (e.g., Tai chi) were effective [32]. A 2023 systematic review of exercise for sleep in older adults *with chronic health conditions* (e.g., osteoarthritis, mobility problems, cognitive impairment) and different living situations (e.g., community, assisted living facilities, nursing homes), found small improvements in objective sleep measures in response to various interventions: yoga, walking, cycling, pilates, or resistance bands [34]. A gap remains regarding the best exercise approaches for older adults with chronic health conditions with sleep problems.

Cognition

The incidence of dementia increases with each decade, from about 10% for people aged 65 years and older to 35% for those 90 years of older, in the USA [35]. Dementia produces relentless declines in mental, physical, and emotional function, with concomitant caregiver strain and high health care costs. The underlying causes of most types of dementia are unknown, which has complicated the search for effective prevention and treatment. However, there is a clear association between vascular disease risk factors—hypertension, DM2, hyperlipidemias, smoking—and the most common dementias: Alzheimer's and vascular dementia. Given the benefits of exercise for these risk factors, many observational and intervention trials of exercise, for prevention and palliation (i.e., slowing cognitive and functional loss) have been conducted.

Epidemiological studies show a strong inverse association with exercise and Alzheimer's and vascular dementias, with a reduced risk of nearly 30% with greater leisure time physical activities, particularly for higher intensity activities [3]. Small trials in older adults suggest that exercise may reduce the risk of cognitive decline, with varied exercise modes, subjects, and outcomes measures [3]. If future, well-designed, larger studies show success in preventing cognitive declines, this could be a potent stimulus for many older adults to get moving.

In terms of slowing the course or improving function in dementia, intervention trials show "promise" according to a 2015 Cochrane Collaboration review [36]. Evidence supports improvements in physical function and ADLs, but is inconclusive regarding cognition and caregiver burden, which are also critical outcomes. A 2022 systematic review and meta-analysis of exercise intervention trials in dementia, from any cause, showed small improvements in cognition, which were larger with regimen adherence and did not differ by type of dementia [37]. No conclusions about preferred type of exercise were possible [37]. The current dementia medications are limited to palliative (i.e., slowing progression) effects or have highly toxic side effects while also palliative. In comparison, exercise is safe and may have physical and ADL function payoffs.

Cancer

Many cancers increase with age and appear due to underlying aging processes (see Chap. 1). Treatments such as surgery and medications are often associated with loss of appetite and fatigue, which in older adults usually means weight loss—primarily muscle loss—accompanied by decreases in strength, endurance, and function [3]. Epidemiologic studies find that physical activity appears to have a protective effect against colon cancer, breast cancer, endometrial cancer, and prostate cancer. Patients who are more active with breast and colon cancer have better survival: almost twice the survival rate as those who are not physically active [3].

In addition to mortality effects, numerous trials have demonstrated benefits of exercise on physical outcomes, such as strength and fitness, in cancer patients. Other studies and meta-analyses have examined exercise effects on cancer-related symptoms of fatigue, well-being, depression, sleep, emotional well-being, and quality of life, with positive results limited primarily to fatigue reduction [3, 38]. The interventions studied are varied with combinations of high-intensity aerobic and resistance exercises, relaxation techniques, and/or massage. A few small studies have examined exercise programs for cachexia associated with cancer, without positive findings [39].

As with other exercise interventions, the program must be tailored to the older adult's baseline physical capacity and other health conditions, with special attention to the patient's immunological status and infection risk, when appropriate.

Frailty and Sarcopenia

Frailty is an age-related clinical syndrome with declines in several bodily functions and overall physiologic reserve. There are different definitions or frailty scores in use. The "phenotype" definition includes having three or more of five symptoms: unintentional weight loss (10 or more pounds within the past year), muscle loss and weakness, fatigue or sense of exhaustion, slow walking speed, and low physical activity. Detecting frailty in older adults has skyrocketed in importance due to many studies revealing frailty to be a critical risk factor for poor outcomes, including mortality, with stresses such as infection, surgery, or cancer treatment [40].

Sarcopenia is a syndrome of accelerated muscle wasting, with low muscle mass, and either low muscle strength or low physical performance. It can occur in persons of any weight, including obese persons, and is associated with poor outcomes. A sedentary lifestyle may lead to sarcopenia, and sarcopenia can be a precursor to frailty.

As older adults with frailty or sarcopenia are at high risk for functional decline, falls, fractures, hospitalizations, and death, studies testing prevention and treatment approaches are a high priority. Exercise and good nutrition appear important for prevention and treatment of both syndromes. A comprehensive 2020 systematic review and meta-analysis concluded that interventions using combinations of resistance, endurance, and balance, and overall physical activity appear to prevent frailty, with too few studies examining sarcopenia prevention for conclusions [41].

For treatment of older adults with frailty or sarcopenia, evidence suggests improvement from resistance exercises in early but not later stages (i.e., higher scores) of frailty and sarcopenia [42]. This finding should encourage early recognition of this syndrome and interventions by health professionals. A 2021 systematic review concluded that, while comparing studies was marred by differing frailty definitions, mixed (aerobic and muscle-strengthening), muscle-strengthening, mobilization and rehabilitation, or aerobic activities all improved markers of mobility, function, and cognition, in pre-frail (low scores) and frail individuals [40].

While the causes of frailty and sarcopenia may be complex and multifactorial, it appears highly likely that exercise plays a critical role in the prevention and treatment of frailty and sarcopenia.

Quality of Life, Successful Aging, and Resilience

Health professionals' and older adults' descriptions of a high quality of life or successful aging do not always align. Traditionally, the medical definition has focused on the absence of disease, "lack of chronic diseases, physical disabilities, and risk factors for disease in older age, as well as good mental health, cognitive function, and social engagement" [1]. The World Health Organization defines "healthy aging" as a "process of developing and maintaining the functional ability that will enable older people to do the things that matter to them" [1]. An extensive scoping review found that older adults valued meaningful relationships, positive attitudes, and adapting to physical changes, as well as being independent, mentally intact, and physically active [43].

These aspirations for aging converge on the ability to maintain cognitive health and functional independence. Exercise is essential for achieving the latter and plays a key role in the former, through effects on cardiovascular, cerebrovascular, and other diseases. Yet very few older adults exercise at levels to achieve their goals of successful aging. Some are entirely sedentary and risk frailty, with impaired resilience at the onset of any new stress.

Health care professionals alone may not solve this paradox, but as relatively trusted experts, they can communicate the astounding array of benefits from exercise to older adults at every interaction. Exercise is medicine: it is often more effective and safer than medications for preventing and treating many conditions that are common in—and feared by—older adults. Indeed, exercise is the "anti-aging pill."

Case: Part 2

Mr. and Mrs. Sampson's daughter tells her parents about how regular exercise can prevent or improve many diseases and conditions seen in older adults. She tells her mother that exercise can reduce the risk of osteoporosis, relieve osteoarthritis pain, treat depression, and help to prevent cognitive decline. She also tells them that exercise reduces cardiovascular risks, including heart attacks, and can improve balance and strength to prevent falls. She tells her father that exercise is key to reducing his risk of diabetes as well as managing his weight. Moreover, his function and energy level can be improved through exercise. Mrs. and Mrs. are very impressed and decide to investigate local programs at the Senior Center. Their daughter reminds them to "start low and go slow!"

References

1. Szychowska A, Drygas W. Physical activity as a determinant of successful aging: a narrative review article. Aging Clin Exp Res. 2022;34:1209–14.
2. Izquierdo M, Fiatarone SM. Promoting resilience in the face of ageing and disease: The central role of exercise and physical activity. Ageing Res Rev. 2023;88:101940.
3. Pedersen BK, Saltin B. Exercise as medicine - evidence for prescribing exercise as therapy in 26 different chronic diseases. Scand J Med Sci Sports. 2015;25(Suppl 3):1–72.
4. Exercise is medicine. https://www.exerciseismedicine.org/. Accessed 2 August 2023.
5. Izquierdo M, Merchant RA, Morley JE, Anker SD, Aprahamian I, Arai H, et al. International exercise recommendations in older adults (ICFSR): expert consensus guidelines. J Nutr Health Aging. 2021;25(7):824–53.
6. WHO guidelines on physical activity and sedentary behavior. https://apps.who.int/iris/bitstream/handle/10665/336656/9789240015128-eng.pdf?sequence=1&isAllowed=y. Accessed 2 August 2023.
7. CDC benefits of exercise. https://www.cdc.gov/physicalactivity/basics/older_adults/index.htm. Accessed 2 August 2023.
8. NHS benefits of exercise. https://www.nhs.uk/live-well/exercise/exercise-health-benefits/. Accessed 2 August 2023.
9. Idland G, Rydwik E, Småstuen MC, Bergland A. Predictors of mobility in community-dwelling women aged 85 and older. Disabil Rehabil. 2013;35(11):881–7.
10. Sjölund B-M, Wimo A, Engström M, von Strauss E. Incidence of ADL disability in older persons, physical activities as a protective factor and the need for informal and formal care – results from the SNAC-N project. PLoS One. 2015;10(9):e0138901.
11. Langhammer B, Bergland A, Rydwik E. The importance of physical activity exercise among older people. Biomed Res Int. 2018;2018:7856823.
12. Okamae A, Ogawa T, Makizako H, Matsumoto D, Ishigaki T, Kamiya M, et al. Efficacy of therapeutic exercise on activities of daily living and cognitive function among older residents in long-term care facilities: a systematic review and meta-analysis of randomized

controlled trials. Arch Phys Med Rehabil. 2023;104(5):812–23. https://doi.org/10.1016/j. apmr.2022.11.002. PMID: 36574530.

13. Treacy D, Hassett L, Schurr K, Fairhall NJ, Cameron ID, Sherrington C. Mobility training for increasing mobility and functioning in older people with frailty. Cochrane Database Syst Rev. 2022;6(6):CD010494. https://doi.org/10.1002/14651858.CD010494.pub2. PMID: 35771806.
14. Roberts CE, Phillips LH, Cooper CL, Gray S, Allan JL. Effect of different types of physical activity on activities of daily living in older adults: systematic review and meta-analysis. J Aging Phys Act. 2017;25(4):653–70.
15. Zhao M, Veeranki SP, Magnussen CG, Xi B. Recommended physical activity and all cause and cause specific mortality in US adults: prospective cohort study. BMJ. 2020;370:m2031. https:// doi.org/10.1136/bmj.m2031. PMID: 32611588.
16. Kujala UM. Is physical activity a cause of longevity? It is not as straightforward as some would believe. A critical analysis. Br J Sports Med. 2018;52(14):914–8.
17. López-Bueno R, Ahmadi M, Stamatakis S et al. Prospective associations of different combinations of aerobic and muscle-strengthening activity with all-cause, cardiovascular, and cancer mortality. JAMA Intern Med. 2023. https://doi.org/10.1001/jamainternmed.2023.3093.
18. CDC Still Going Strong. https://www.cdc.gov/stillgoingstrong/olderadults/index.html. Accessed 2 August 2023.
19. Sherrington C, Fairhall NJ, Wallbank GK, Tiedemann A, Michaleff ZA, Howard K, Clemson L, Hopewell S, Lamb SE. Exercise for preventing falls in older people living in the community. Cochrane Database Syst Rev. 2019;1(1):CD012424.
20. Montero-Odasso MM, Kamkar N, Pieruccini-Faria F, Osman A, Sarquis-Adamson Y, Close J, et al. Evaluation of clinical practice guidelines on fall prevention and management for older adults. A systematic review. JAMA Netw Open. 2021;4(12):e2138911. https://doi.org/10.1001/jamanetworkopen.2021.38911.
21. Brooke-Wavell K, Skelton DA, Barker KL, Clark EM, De Biase S, Arnold S, Paskins Z, Robinson KR, Lewis RM, Tobias JH, Ward KA, Whitney J, Leyland S. Strong, steady and straight: UK consensus statement on physical activity and exercise for osteoporosis. Br J Sports Med. 2022;56(15):837–46.
22. Pinheiro MB, Oliveira J, Bauman A, et al. Evidence on physical activity and osteoporosis prevention for people aged 65+ years: a systematic review to inform the WHO guidelines on physical activity and sedentary behaviour. Int J Behav Nutr Phys Act. 2020;17:150.
23. Franklin BA, Thompson PD, Al-Zaiti SS, et al. Exercise-related acute cardiovascular events and potential deleterious adaptations following long-term exercise training: placing the risks into perspective–an update: a scientific statement from the American Heart Association. Circulation. 2020;141:e705–36.
24. Barbiellini Amidei C, Trevisan C, Dotto M, et al. Association of physical activity trajectories with major cardiovascular diseases in elderly people. Heart. 2022;108:360–6.
25. Dibben GO, Faulkner J, Oldridge N, Rees K, Thompson DR, Zwisler A-D, Taylor RS. Exercise-based cardiac rehabilitation for coronary heart disease: a meta-analysis. Eur Heart J. 2023;44(6):452–69.
26. Kumar KR, Pina IL. Cardiac rehabilitation in older adults: new options. Clin Cardiol. 2020;43(2):163–70. https://doi.org/10.1002/clc.23296. Epub 2019 Dec 11. PMID: 31823400; PMCID: PMC7021654.
27. Edwards JJ, Deenmamode AHP, Griffiths M, et al. Exercise training and resting blood pressure: a large-scale pairwise and network meta-analysis of randomised controlled trials. Br J Sports Med. 2023;57(20):1317–26.
28. Lane R, Harwood A, Watson L, Leng GC. Exercise for intermittent claudication. Cochrane Database Syst Rev. 2017;12(12):CD000990. https://doi.org/10.1002/14651858.CD000990. pub4. PMID: 29278423.
29. McCarthy B, Casey D, Devane D, Murphy K, Murphy E, Lacasse Y. Pulmonary rehabilitation for chronic obstructive pulmonary disease. Cochrane Database Syst Rev. 2015;2:CD003793.
30. Luck-Sikorski C, Stein J, Heilmann K, Maier W, Kaduszkiewicz H, Scherer M, et al. Treatment preferences for depression in the elderly. Int Psychogeriatr. 2017;29(3):389–98.

31. Cooney GM, Dwan K, Greig CA, Lawlor DA, Rimer J, Waugh FR, McMurdo M, Mead GE. Exercise for depression. Cochrane Database Syst Rev. 2013;9:CD004366.
32. Vanderlinden J, Boen F, van Uffelen JG. Effects of physical activity programs on sleep outcomes in older adults: a systematic review. Int J Behav Nutr Phys Act. 2020;17(1):11. https://doi.org/10.1186/s12966-020-0913-3.
33. Xie Y, Liu S, Chen X-J, Yu H-H, Yang Y, Wang W. Effects of exercise on sleep quality and insomnia in adults: a systematic review and meta-analysis of randomized controlled trials. Front Psych. 2021;12:664499.
34. Solis-Navarro L, Masot O, Torres-Castro R, Otto-Yáñez M, Fernández-Jané C, Solà-Madurell M, Coda A, Cyrus-Barker E, Sitjà-Rabert M, Pérez LM. Effects on sleep quality of physical exercise programs in older adults: a systematic review and meta-analysis. Clocks Sleep. 2023;5(2):152–66.
35. Manly JJ, Jones RN, Langa KM, Ryan LH, Levine DA, McCammon R, Heeringa SG, Weir D. Estimating the prevalence of dementia and mild cognitive impairment in the US. The 2016 health and retirement study harmonized cognitive assessment protocol project. JAMA Neurol. 2022;79(12):1242–9.
36. Forbes D, Forbes SC, Blake CM, Thiessen EJ, Forbes S. Exercise programs for people with dementia. Cochrane Database Syst Rev. 2015;4:CD006489.
37. Balbim GM, Falck RS, Barha CK, Starkey SY, Bullock A, Davis JC, Liu-Ambrose T. Effects of exercise training on the cognitive function of older adults with different types of dementia: a systematic review and meta-analysis. Br J Sports Med. 2022. https://doi.org/10.1136/bjsports-2021-104955.
38. Loughney LA, West MA, Kemp GJ, Grocott MPW, Jack S. Exercise interventions for people undergoing multimodal cancer treatment that includes surgery. Cochrane Database Syst Rev. 2018;12:CD012280.
39. Grande AJ, Silva V, Sawaris Neto L, Teixeira Basmage JP, Peccin MS, Maddocks M. Exercise for cancer cachexia in adults. Cochrane Database Syst Rev. 2021;3:CD010804.
40. Racey M, Ali MU, Sherifali D, Fitzpatrick-Lewis D, Lewis R, Jovkovic M, Bouchard DR, Giguère A, Holroyd-Leduc J, Tang A, Gramlich L, Keller H, Prorok J, Kim P, Lorbergs A, Muscedere J. Effectiveness of physical activity interventions in older adults with frailty or prefrailty: a systematic review and meta-analysis. CMAJ Open. 2021;9(3):728–43.
41. Oliveira JS, Pinheiro MB, Fairhall N, Walsh S, Chesterfield Franks T, Kwok W, Bauman A, Sherrington C. Evidence on physical activity and the prevention of frailty and sarcopenia among older people: a systematic review to inform the World Health Organization physical activity guidelines. J Phys Act Health. 2020;17(12):1247–58. https://doi.org/10.1123/jpah.2020-0323.
42. Talar K, Hernández-Belmonte A, Vetrovsky T, Steffl M, Kałamacka E, Courel-Ibáñez J. Benefits of resistance training in early and late stages of frailty and sarcopenia: a systematic review and meta-analysis of randomized controlled studies. J Clin Med. 2021;10:1630.
43. Teater B, Chonody JM. How do older adults define successful aging? A scoping review. Int J Aging Hum Dev. 2020;91(4):599–625.

Chapter 3
Risks of Exercise in Older Adults

Joseph C. Watso and Joseph D. Vondrasek

Key Points
- The leading exercise risk is musculoskeletal injury (sprains, fractures, etc.) and the most significant risk is acute death, often of cardiovascular origin
- Much of this elevated risk in older adults can be mitigated through a careful and conservative progression from inactive to highly physically active
- Education for risk mitigation strategies can reduce the risks of exercise
- With the use of proper risk mitigation strategies, the majority of common diseases are not associated with significantly greater health risks from exercise
- Some clinical conditions, such as end-stage renal disease, will require careful exercise supervision to manage exercise risks

Case: Part 1
George is a retired 75-year-old man with occasional knee pain due to osteoarthritis, hypertension, hyperlipidemia, and a heart attack 10 years ago when his hypertension and hyperlipidemia were first discovered. He used to bowl, but stopped at the time of his heart attack and admits he's a "couch potato." His weight has crept up along with his hemoglobin A1C, which his doctor says can lead to type 2 diabetes. His medical conditions are under excellent control with aspirin, a lipid-lowering drug, and two antihypertensive medicines. George knows that exercising would be good for his health, but he worries that exercise could make his knees worse and give him a heart attack.

J. C. Watso (✉) · J. D. Vondrasek
Cardiovascular and Applied Physiology Laboratory, Department of Health, Nutrition, and Food Sciences, Florida State University, Tallahassee, FL, USA
e-mail: jwatso@fsu.edu

Table 3.1 Acute cardiovascular risks of exercise in adults [4]	1 sudden cardiac death per 1,500,000 vigorous exercise bouts in men
	1 sudden cardiac death per 36,500,000 h of moderate-to-vigorous intensity exercise in women
	1 death per 2,897,057 person-hours at YMCA gyms
	1 cardiac arrest per 500,000 runner-hours
	1 sudden cardiac death per 714,286 runner-hours
	1 cardiovascular event per 1667 symptom-limited cardiopulmonary exercise tests

Should Your Patient Exercise?

There are multiple resources available when considering exercise risks. The *Exercise and Screening for You* (EASY) tool is a helpful online resource for risk assessment in older adults and matches activities to individual needs [1]. For all adults, the *Physical Activity Readiness Questionnaire for Everyone* (PAR-Q+) is another questionnaire about individual exercise risks [2]. The initial seven questions cover general health. For those with existing conditions, ten additional items can serve as discussion points for specific conditions (e.g., cancer, cancer type, current therapy regimen, etc.) [2]. The American Heart Association argues that pre-participation exercise testing with ECG monitoring is unnecessary for older adults without exertional (exercise-induced) symptoms [3]. Higher risk individuals, such as those with heart failure, should undergo ECG monitoring during a pre-participation exercise test. In some cases, echocardiographic studies may help with risk stratification for selecting safe exercise intensities. This approach can mitigate the most dangerous risks of exercise, those related to acute adverse cardiovascular events: sudden cardiac death and myocardial infarction [4]. Of note, these serious risks are highest during vigorous exercise in sedentary adults (Table 3.1). Importantly, these risks decline substantially with exercise training [3].

Where Should Your Patient Exercise?

For those ready to initiate exercise, there are risks associated with certain environments. One obvious example is high crime areas. If it is not possible to avoid such environments, older adults should exercise with a group during the daytime or in well-lit areas. Exercising on sidewalks, walking/biking paths, or bike lanes can add an audience of traffic, to avoid being alone. However, traffic comes with risks as well. For example, a bike lane with a physical barrier is much safer than a white line on the pavement separating the biker from vehicle traffic. Thus, older adults should aim for low or slow vehicle traffic areas. For those who prefer parks, look for shock-absorbing surfaces and well-maintained areas without obstacles, such as objects lying around (tripping hazards) or holes in the ground. Finally, for outdoor sports, facilities with anchored and padded goals, goal posts, and fences are preferable to prevent injuries.

When exercising outdoors, a major consideration is the ambient environment's UV radiation, temperature, altitude, and/or pollution. For example, while exercise reduces the risk of nearly all types of cancer, exercise is associated with *higher* skin cancer risk, particularly in those with lower skin pigmentation [5]. Thus, during high UV conditions, older adults should prioritize sun protection via sunscreen, lightweight clothing coverage, or shade. One freely available tool is *UVLens* (www. uvlens.com). This website and free phone application provide personalized suggestions for safety in the sun.

Related to UV exposure, heat is another key concern for older adults. Older adults have poorer thermoregulation because of reduced blood flow redistribution from the core to the skin (for cooling) and reduced sweating (for cooling). Older adults also have reduced thirst sensation which can further contribute to increased core temperature and lead to dehydration-related dizziness and falls [6]. Moreover, older adults have greater increases in body temperature in extreme heat, compared to younger adults, even when water intake is controlled [7]. Increased core temperature can strain the cardiovascular system (e.g., needing to increase blood flow to the skin to cool down) and increase the risk of adverse cardiovascular and non-cardiovascular events. Therefore, older adults should avoid exercising in extreme heat when possible and have a plan to consume fluids to remain hydrated.

However, cold also poses risks for older adults. Snow shoveling after major snowstorms is associated with high cardiovascular event risk [3]. The cause is likely a combination of three factors. First, snow shoveling increases the metabolic rate to about 5–7 times higher than rest. This is of concern for some older adults because, on average, a 60–69 years old has a *peak* exercise capacity of only 6–7 times that of rest [8, 9]. Thus, older persons shoveling snow are likely operating very close to their peak exercise capacity. Second, many inactive individuals choose to shovel snow and the relative risk of a heart attack is nearly 50 times higher in a sedentary adult than one who exercises vigorously (equivalent to an intensity that evokes substantial increases in heart rate and breathing [≥60% of peak exercise capacity] 5 or more days per week) [3]. This statistic drives home the imperative to start exercising at a low level and slowly ramp up exercise training, to reduce the risk of an exercise-induced cardiovascular event. In short, being untrained increases risks. The third contributing factor is that in cold temperatures, cold-induced vasoconstriction may lower the threshold of chest pain to a lower rate pressure product (heart rate × systolic blood pressure).

Exercise during the first day at high altitude (>4200 feet) can increase the risk of a cardiovascular event from the novel stress of slight hypoxia [3]. Thus, it is best to acclimate for at least one night before exercising, even in healthy adults of all ages.

Air pollution poses additional problems for older adults. In severe cases of air pollution, now often seen as a result of distant wildfires, older adults and others with health conditions are warned to remain indoors [10]. Airway reactions to pollutants, increased cardiovascular stress, and mucosal irritation can lead to exacerbation of underlying conditions. Planning to exercise indoors during times of high heat, cold, and pollution is increasingly important.

Indoors, equipment such as free weights, treadmills, and other machines can expand exercise options for older adults. Individuals with little or no experience with equipment and safe movements are at increased risk of injury. Even those with prior gym experience may realize that their previous form was poor. With aging, poor position can produce pain or increase injuries due to the use of vulnerable body positions. Conversely, the form may be correct, but age-related changes, such as reduced balance or range of motion, make some movements (e.g., overhead free weights) unsafe. Generally, using weight or aerobic machines with fixed ranges of motion (e.g., seated triceps extension or an elliptical machine) will reduce injury risk relative to free-weight movements or open aerobic machines (e.g., overhead dumbbell shoulder press or a treadmill). Another approach is training with a spotter, preferably one who is experienced, such as an American College of Sports Medicine-certified trainer, who will monitor for safe use of free-weight movements (e.g., kettlebell goblet squats). Injury risks are also reduced by using the safety features of certain devices such as holding the handrails and clipping the safety key onto clothing when using a treadmill.

Water exercise is highly recommended for those with joint problems, such as osteoarthritis, as well as for older adults with current fall risks. However, drowning risk must be minimized. This will be reduced through safety instruction and ensuring supervision with a lifeguard.

In summary, risks of outdoor and indoor exercise can be minimized greatly with attention to outdoor conditions, use of equipment safety features, and/or instruction for new activities.

How Should Your Patient Exercise?

The most common injuries in older adults are strains (muscle or tendon) and sprains (ligaments) [11]. Warming up before and cooling down after exercise to reduce these risks is discussed in Chap. 11. The next most common injuries are fractures in the upper and lower extremities. Falling due to loss of balance and reduced bone health are the major causes of fractures, thus, attention to balance is essential in planning safe exercise for older persons. For those with balance issues, poor bone health, or who are new to exercising, working with a trainer can reduce the risk of injury. For all older adults, starting at low levels and slowly increasing effort is recommended (see Chap. 6). Pickleball and tennis are among the highest injury risk sports [12, 13], yet many adults enjoy these activities. Individuals will need to balance personal preference and exercise enjoyment against the risks of injury and potential resulting functional loss. Forced sedentary behavior after a major adverse event, such as a fracture, can result in permanent effects on function. Therefore, exercise selection should consider the second-order consequences of high-risk sports participation, with the ultimate goal of staying physically active for life.

Disease-Specific Considerations

Osteoporosis and Conditions Affecting Balance

The risk of falling is higher when the terrain is difficult, such as hiking on a trail or walking on steep slopes. Also, those who have difficulty balancing, have osteoporosis (low bone density), and/or decreased leg muscle strength have a higher risk of falls resulting in a fracture. To reduce injuries, older adults can select a treadmill with handles, rather than walking over the ground, for initial exercise. This controlled walking can improve leg strength and balance exercises can be added later, to include overground walking. Additionally, for resistance training, one can use machines with built-in weight pulleys rather than free weights, where the risk of injury, due to unsafe ranges of motion, is higher.

Adults affected by Parkinson's disease, multiple sclerosis, spinal cord injuries, or stroke history need to carefully select exercises. For an adult with Parkinson's disease, a step-through (lower frame, such as near the floor) stationary bike should be selected rather than a step-over (waist-high frame) bike. Additionally, an arm ergometer may be used for upper body endurance exercise. Based on balance-related high risk of falling and related injuries, these individuals should avoid pickleball, tennis, and other sports requiring rapid changes in body position [14].

Adults with orthostatic disorders, in which the blood pressure decreases with moving to an upright position, can reduce the risk of falls by making postural changes (e.g., sit-to-stand) slowly and by staying well-hydrated when exercising [15].

Cardiovascular Diseases

Irrespective of underlying cardiovascular disease, age increases risk for cardiovascular-related complications during exercise.

Heart Failure

In heart failure, the heart cannot meet increased metabolic demands which leads to shortness of breath and exercise intolerance [16]. Despite a lowered exercise capacity, current evidence suggests that the risk of adverse events during exercise for patients with heart failure is low and exercise improves quality of life [17]. The most common adverse events for these patients are post-exercise hypotension, atrial and ventricular arrhythmias, and worsening of symptoms such as dyspnea. Given these risks, it is recommended that patients with heart failure start exercising under supervision to improve confidence and perceived efficacy, and reduce risks, before exercising independently in an exercise center or at home.

Hypertension

Exercise can reduce blood pressure and is a first line treatment for hypertension. Risks to consider during exercise include an exaggerated blood pressure response and subsequent acute adverse cardiovascular events [18]. During exercise that involves a Valsalva maneuver (expiration against a closed glottis), the acute spike in blood pressure may produce dizziness and fainting. Alpha-blockers, used for hypertension and other conditions, can cause hypotension [19]. Thus, additional caution should be used when starting exercise for individuals taking these medications. Beta-blockers are used to treat hypertension, angina, heart failure, and other conditions [20]. A key physiological effect of these medications is a lower heart rate and blood pressure, at rest and during exercise, which will reduce maximum exercise heart rate and capacity. The initiation of beta-blocker or other rate-lowering medications may require lowering the prescribed heart rate for a given exercise intensity. Alternatively, rather than heart rate, intensity can be gauged via rate of perceived effort or breathlessness. There is also evidence suggesting that taking beta-blockers increases the risk of heat-related illness and heat stroke, thus, patients taking these medications should closely monitor ambient conditions [21]. Treatment with beta-blockers may also affect glycemic control and hypoglycemic symptoms, which means it is important to monitor for symptoms of hypo- and hyperglycemia before, during, and after exercise [22, 23].

Blow flow restriction training is a popular exercise technique used during resistance training and rehabilitation, but poses risks to many older adults [24]. The goal is to attain the benefits of high-intensity resistance or aerobic exercise (i.e., muscle growth) by mimicking the cellular environment of vigorous exercise. This is accomplished by restricting blood flow and increasing blood metabolite build-up. This flow restriction technique augments the exercise pressor reflex which increases blood pressure and sympathetic nervous system activity; this can raise the likelihood of a cardiovascular event. Individuals with cardiovascular conditions—heart failure, peripheral artery disease, and hypertension—need careful monitoring and may need to avoid blood flow restriction training.

Stroke

The incidence of stroke or cerebrovascular events increases with age. Regular physical activity is integral to secondary stroke prevention [25]. Changes in physical, emotional, and cognitive function after a cerebrovascular accident vary with the size and location of the affected area within the brain, with varying exercise risks. Exercise monitoring should include attention to mood, motivation, frustration, and confusion [4]. Even after completing a rehabilitation program with a physical and occupational therapist, there may be residual decrements in functional capacity, balance, and speech. An impairment to balance or stability translates to a higher risk of falls and injury during exercise. If the older adult suffers from speech problems post-stroke, there may be difficulty communicating pain, discomfort, and other symptoms. Thus, exercise supervisors need to remain attentive during exercise for these patients [4]. Given the array of outcomes for patients after a stroke, a full pre-participation screening and medical health evaluation is essential to ensure medical stability and create safe exercise plans.

Pulmonary Embolism

Although pulmonary embolus can present significant challenges for older adults planning to exercise, decrements in physical capacity may be related more to general deconditioning than pulmonary embolus effects [26]. After a pulmonary embolus, increased fatigue after exercise is more likely if the patient had pre-morbid fatigue with activities of daily living. Symptoms of dyspnea, dizziness, chest pain, and psychological stress (anxiety and problems with sleep) occur after a pulmonary embolus, thus, monitoring for these symptoms is important when initiating exercise [27]. Starting low and going slow during exercise is essential for these individuals, with attention to vital signs (pulse, blood pressure, oxygenation) as well as symptoms [26].

Arthritis, Osteoarthritis, and Joint Replacements

Arthritis

Osteoarthritis and rheumatoid arthritis are the most common types of arthritis, with osteoarthritis being especially common in older adults. Arthritis is the second leading cause of disability and 1 in 2 adults in the USA and Canada have arthritis [28–30]. The American College of Rheumatology and other groups strongly recommend exercise as part of arthritis treatment, since patients with arthritis who remain active report less pain, improved sleep, and better function when performing activities of daily living [31, 32]. Unfortunately, this message has not reached some patients with arthritis and health professionals, who believe exercise, especially weight-bearing exercise (resistance training, walking, etc.), will exacerbate joint damage and worsen symptoms of pain and fatigue [33]. However, there is little additional risk during exercise for adults with arthritis. Table 3.2 contains some exercise considerations and mitigation strategies for older adults with arthritis.

Joint Replacement: Knee and Hip

Replacement joint surgeries increase with age and are often related to osteoarthritis. About 7 million US adults have had a knee or hip replacement surgery [34]. Assuming the older adult has completed an adequate rehabilitation program with physical and occupational therapists, there is minimal additional risk posed by a

Table 3.2 Exercise risks, considerations, and mitigation strategies for adults with arthritis

Risk	Reason	Mitigation strategy
Moderate pain or soreness with exercise	It is not uncommon to have pain during and/or immediately after exercise—especially during a new activity	Reassurance that it is not dangerous to have some pain with exercise and, as the activity becomes more familiar, the pain may decrease Avoid exercising during peak pain and exercise while the pain relief from medications is highest If pain lasts more than 2 h after exercise, consider decreasing the intensity during the next session
Injury	Patients with arthritis commonly have diminished functional capacity so rushing into vigorous exercise may lead to injuries	Begin exercising at a low intensity and slowly increase intensity as the person progresses
Discouragement	A person with arthritis may assume that they should progress at a rate faster than they can. The smaller-than-expected improvement may lead to discouragement	Before starting an exercise program, remind the person that progress may be slow at first, but this is expected Even small improvements are still improvements Remind the person to focus on their exercise journey and encourage them to avoid comparing their progress to others' progress
Pain during specific movements	Depending on the arthritis presentation, pain may occur during specific movements	Find an exercise that works for a similar joint or muscle group but causes less pain or no pain For example, if squatting causes pain in the knee, try switching to the leg extension machine as a quadriceps exercise or pool walking

thoughtful exercise program. After a total knee replacement, risk during exercise increases with exercise intensity, because of the increased joint loads. Low-to-intermediate intensity activities (cycling, swimming, golf) have a lower risk of prosthesis complications, such as joint wear, osteolysis, and prosthetic failure, as compared to higher-intensity activities (jogging, water skiing, soccer) [35]. However, it is important to consider the person's previous training, because risk during technical sports activities is lower for those with prior training [36]. Balance and sensorimotor function may not be fully restored after joint replacement surgery unless there is a sustained focus on these functions. If not, there may be an increased risk of falls [35]. After a total hip replacement, a primary early concern is joint dislocation, particularly with internal rotation of the hip. Post-replacement rehabilitation programs typically include patient education regarding the prevention of hip joint dislocation. In addition, the risk of dislocation is very low and, with recent advances in surgical techniques, this risk has decreased further [37].

As discussed, there may be minimal risks for adults with arthritis, but existing comorbidities, such as obesity, diabetes, or heart disease, will contribute risk [29]. These conditions are more common among adults with arthritis and will confer independent risks that must be considered in counseling for exercise. Overall, the benefits of exercise for older adults with arthritis far outweigh the risks.

Metabolic and Renal Diseases

Metabolic Syndrome

Metabolic syndrome is a constellation of concurrent conditions (elevated blood pressure, elevated blood glucose, dyslipidemia, high waist circumference) that increase the risk of cardiovascular and other diseases. Based on the current evidence, it is unclear whether this syndrome is a unique pathological entity. Hence, the relevant risks of exercise are discussed separately for each condition.

Diabetes Mellitus

In the USA, 1 in 3 adults over 65 years old has diabetes mellitus [38]. Changes in blood glucose and heat intolerance are key risks during exercise associated with diabetes. Low blood sugar, or hypoglycemia, is a potential risk before and after exercise for patients with type 1 (T1DM) and type 2 Diabetes mellitus (T2DM), but it is more common among those with T1DM. Hypoglycemia before exercise increases the risk of severe hypoglycemia during exercise. Most post-exercise hypoglycemia occurs 6–15 h after exercise but can occur up to 48 h later [39]. Conversely, hyperglycemia may occur after high-intensity exercise (T1DM) because of elevated glucagon, epinephrine, and other changes. This is a natural and expected change, but without an adequate insulin response, the circulating glucose will not be appropriately sequestered into cells [39]. Hence, proper glucose monitoring and management are essential to minimize deleterious changes in blood glucose before, during, and after exercise, particularly for those with T1DM.

There is a potential increased risk of heat-related illness among persons with diabetes if they have developed impaired skin blood flow and neuropathy, leading to the decreased ability to sweat and dissipate heat [40]. Also, in the setting of hyperglycemia, subsequent polyuria can lead to dehydration and further dysregulation of core temperature [40]. When individuals with diabetes begin an exercise program, it may be best to start indoors in a temperature-controlled environment to avoid the risks of heat-related illness, in locales with high ambient temperatures.

Dyslipidemia

About 30% of adults in the USA have dyslipidemia. Combined treatment of dyslipidemia with statin medications and exercise produces better outcomes than exercise or statins alone [41]. Fortunately, there is minimal risk during exercise independent of comorbidities, for these patients. Statins are among the most commonly taken prescription medications in the world and thus well-studied. Persons taking statins may note muscle pain or myalgias [42]. However, studies have found that when comparing patients who are blinded and unblinded to statin use, the patients who are unblinded report muscle-related adverse events at a higher rate, which suggests patient or physician expectations are a strong driver of these symptoms. Similarly, re-challenging persons with prior complaints of statin-related muscle pains, in a blinded fashion, shows very low symptom recurrence [43].

Chronic Kidney Disease

Fifteen percent of US adults have chronic kidney disease (CKD) and the incidence is expected to rise with the growing prevalence of obesity and diabetes. Regular exercise is viewed positively by patients with CKD and physicians, but exercise is not always implemented [44]. Comorbidities such as diabetes, hypertension, and obesity are common among this population, but once risks related to these and other conditions, such as cardiovascular disease, have been addressed, there are a few additional risks for patients with CKD. First, patients with CKD are at a higher risk of injuries because of associated bone disease [45]. Also, if a patient is receiving dialysis, there may be fatigue following dialysis; exercising before treatment or between dialysis days may prevent exercise avoidance. Hypotension may occur during treatment and should also be considered when scheduling exercise [46]. If a patient has frequent episodes of hypotension, recumbent biking will be safer than walking on a treadmill, to prevent falls and injuries. Lastly, if a patient is receiving peritoneal dialysis treatment, they may have abdominal excess fluid and/or discomfort which may affect exercise regimens [47].

Respiratory Diseases

Communicable Diseases

Since the COVID-19 pandemic, it is easy to appreciate the risk of respiratory infection transmission in a gym or other group setting. Indoor spaces with many people ventilating more than at rest increase the risk of spreading respiratory infections. Vaccines help to reduce the likelihood of infection and infection severity, thus, when recommending indoor group exercise, immunization discussions are relevant. Opting for off-peak times, less crowded facilities or areas within a facility, and continued germ hygiene (mask usage, hand washing, equipment cleaning) can reduce these risks. Individuals using immunosuppressants or those with existing conditions affecting the immune system should consider indoor risks in comparison to outdoor- or home-based exercise. Most older adults will obtain substantial benefits from a combination of these options, to take account of weather conditions and prevalent respiratory illnesses.

Chronic Obstructive Pulmonary Disease

Chronic obstructive pulmonary disease (COPD) represents diseases of airflow blockage and increased breathing effort. While exercising is safe and effective in COPD, the American Lung Association recommends limiting the intensity and duration of exercise to prevent provoking symptoms, such as shortness of breath [48, 49]. Indeed, the American Lung Association's recommendations for COPD nearly mirror that of the general population, to perform "20–30 min of moderate exercise for 3–4 days a week" [49]. For individuals with greater illness severity, slow pursed lip or belly breathing is recommended during exercise. Moreover, those using supplemental oxygen should continue to use supplemental oxygen during exercise, with adjustments to the flow rate per the prescribing health professional. Older adults with COPD should also avoid isometric and certain high-strain exercises, such as push-ups [50]. Finally, there is a physiological overlap between COPD and obesity regarding breathing mechanics [51]. Specifically, the risk of dyspnea is much higher in individuals with obesity [52]. Similar to asthma, limiting activities when pollution is high or when temperatures are low will reduce symptoms.

Asthma

In asthma, which is due to outflow obstruction from bronchoconstriction, the risks of exercise are low with screening and the use of appropriate prescribed medications [53]. Indeed, exercise training reduces symptoms and improves pulmonary function in persons with asthma [54]. If symptoms arise during exercise, the use of a (rescue) inhaler is often recommended and should be kept available. Older adults with asthma should avoid outdoor activity when air pollution or allergen indices are high and temperatures are low [55]. A scarf or face-covering during cold or dry conditions may reduce discomfort. Also, extended-duration exercise can be avoided if this produces symptoms, with a switch to more frequent, shorter duration exercise [56].

Cancer

Exercise is safe and effective for mortality risk reduction in cancer survivors, particularly for adults with breast, colorectal, or prostate cancer and after hematopoietic stem cell transplantation. Individuals with anemia may report fatigue or shortness of breath. In women exercising after breast cancer treatments, caution for increasing upper body exercise too quickly, as well as protecting an arm at risk of lymphedema, are advised. Wearing well-fitting compression garments during strength training may be recommended.

Exercise trainers or supervisors must understand the effects of each treatment modality, at the individual level, to adjust the exercise program appropriately. For example, expert consensus recommends screening for peripheral neuropathies and musculoskeletal morbidities, secondary to treatment, in patients after cancer treatments [57]. Additionally, those with metastatic bone disease or on hormonal therapy should be assessed for fracture risk before exercise participation. If cancer treatment involves surgery, the patient should delay starting exercise until they are adequately healed, which will vary by surgery and patient. Another example is the need to avoid excessive intra-abdominal pressure (e.g., via the Valsalva maneuver with a heavy lift) in persons following treatment of colon cancer.

In general, individualized recommendations are most appropriate in patients after cancer surgery and other treatments, yet exercise lowers the mortality risk. An excellent resource is the Moving Through Cancer online site that includes cancer-specific assessments for exercise participation and related information [58].

Alzheimer's and Other Dementias

Exercise is safe and may reduce the risk of dementia [59, 60]. The Alzheimer's Society states that "of all the lifestyle changes that have been studied, regular physical exercise appears to be one of the best things that you can do to reduce your risk of getting dementia" [61]. Also, some exercise studies show functional improvement in patients with dementia. However, exercise programs for older adults with dementia may be complicated by memory, language, and other cognitive changes. Supervision is recommended with attention to appropriate exercise attire (e.g., supportive closed-toe shoes), hydration (drinking water before and after exercise), and safe operation of exercise equipment. Moreover, the National Institutes of Aging recommends that individuals with Alzheimer's disease have an Alzheimer's Association ID bracelet with a caregiver's phone number if they walk alone [62, 63]. Finally, for this group, fall prevention concerns need to be considered and mitigated (see section "Osteoporosis and Conditions Affecting Balance").

Conclusion

Exercise is a critical tool to improve both health-span and lifespan. However, older adults have increased risks of exercise-related injuries and death related mainly to existing conditions and medications. Thus, identification and attention to co-morbid conditions is critical. Screening with appropriate tools and a focus on mitigation strategies specific to underlying conditions is essential. These strategies can include working within a healthcare team, such as an oncologist helping an exercise physiologist understand how best to design an exercise program before, during, and after treatment, to reduce exercise risks. For most if not all older adults, being sedentary poses greater risks than exercise.

Case: Part 2

George's clinician thinks that exercise will improve his vascular risks, reduce his chance of developing type 2 diabetes, and likely improve his knee function. Using the EASY and PAR-Q+ tools, George and his clinician evaluate his risks and conclude that he can safely start exercising, without further tests beyond the history and physical exam.

George is glad to hear that his knee pain may improve with exercise, which should also make him stronger, help him lose weight, and improve his cardiovascular health. His clinician tells him to "start low and go slow," and pay attention to hydration and specific symptoms when he should stop exercising and report back, such as breathing too hard to talk, dizziness, chest pain, or knee pain that persists or worsens. He decides to walk daily during good weather, starting at 5 min a day and slowly increasing. Twice a week, and when it is hot, wet, cold, or icy outdoors, he will visit the local Y. He will start with a low level beginner group class with all exercise components, to learn how to use equipment (recumbent bike) and the resistance machines. He feels safe doing this with others and being able to ask questions.

References

1. EASY - Exercise and Screening for You. https://www.easyforyou.info/screening-tool.
2. PAR-Q+. https://www.acsm.org/education-resources/trending-topics-resources/resource-library/detail?id=98750bc1-40c5-44aa-9a08-bdbe7430a3f0.
3. Franklin BA, Thompson PD, Al-Zaiti SS, et al. Exercise-related acute cardiovascular events and potential deleterious adaptations following long-term exercise training: placing the risks into perspective–an update: a scientific statement from the American Heart Association. Circulation. 2020;141(13):e705–36. https://doi.org/10.1161/CIR.0000000000000749.
4. Liguori G, Feito Y, Fountaine C, Roy BA, American College of Sports M. ACSM's guidelines for exercise testing and prescription. 11th ed. Philadelphia: Wolters Kluwer; 2022.
5. Behrens G, Niedermaier T, Berneburg M, Schmid D, Leitzmann MF. Physical activity, cardiorespiratory fitness and risk of cutaneous malignant melanoma: systematic review and meta-analysis. PLoS One. 2018;13(10):e0206087. https://doi.org/10.1371/journal.pone.0206087.
6. Phillips PA, Bretherton M, Risvanis J, Casley D, Johnston C, Gray L. Effects of drinking on thirst and vasopressin in dehydrated elderly men. Am J Phys. 1993;264(5):877–81. https://doi.org/10.1152/ajpregu.1993.264.5.R877.
7. McKenna ZJ, Foster J, Atkins WC, et al. Age alters the thermoregulatory responses to extreme heat exposure with accompanying activities of daily living. J Appl Physiol. 2023;135(2):445–55. https://doi.org/10.1152/japplphysiol.00285.2023.

8. Ainsworth BE, Haskell WL, Herrmann SD, et al. 2011 compendium of physical activities: a second update of codes and MET values. Med Sci Sports Exerc. 2011;43(8):1575–81. https://doi.org/10.1249/MSS.0b013e31821ece12.

9. Peterman JE, Arena R, Myers J, et al. Reference standards for peak rating of perceived exertion during cardiopulmonary exercise testing: data from FRIEND. Med Sci Sports Exerc. 2023;55(1):74–9. https://doi.org/10.1249/mss.0000000000003023.

10. Utendorfer H. Smog and the city: the worsening air pollution in SLC. The Daily Utah Chronicle. https://dailyutahchronicle.com/2021/11/02/smog-city-air-pollution-slc/.

11. Dunsky A, Netz Y. Physical activity and sport in advanced age: is it risky? A summary of data from articles published between 2000-2009. Curr Aging Sci. 2012;5(1):66–71. https://doi.org/10.2174/1874609811205010066.

12. Burfield et al. Phys Ther Sport. 2023;61:1–10.

13. Dhillon et al. Orthop J Sports Med. 2023;11(3):23259671231152900.

14. Weiss H, Dougherty J, DiMaggio C. Non-fatal senior pickleball and tennis-related injuries treated in United States emergency departments, 2010-2019. Inj Epidemiol. 2021;8(1):34. https://doi.org/10.1186/s40621-021-00327-9.

15. Ostrenga S. Managing postural hypotension during exercise. https://www.canr.msu.edu/news/managing_postural_hypotension_during_exercise.

16. Piña IL, Apstein CS, Balady GJ, et al. Exercise and heart failure. Circulation. 2003;107(8):1210–25. https://doi.org/10.1161/01.CIR.0000055013.92097.40.

17. Patti A, Merlo L, Ambrosetti M, Sarto P. Exercise-based cardiac rehabilitation programs in heart failure patients. Heart Fail Clin. 2021;17(2):263–71. https://doi.org/10.1016/j.hfc.2021.01.007.

18. Edwards JJ, Deenmamode AHP, Griffiths M, et al. Exercise training and resting blood pressure: a large-scale pairwise and network meta-analysis of randomised controlled trials. Br J Sports Med. 2023;57(20):1317–26. https://doi.org/10.1136/bjsports-2022-106503.

19. Hiremath S, Ruzicka M, Petrcich W, et al. Alpha-blocker use and the risk of hypotension and hypotension-related clinical events in women of advanced age. Hypertension. 2019;74(3):645–51. https://doi.org/10.1161/HYPERTENSIONAHA.119.13289.

20. do Vale GT, Ceron CS, Gonzaga NA, Simplicio JA, Padovan JC. Three generations of β-blockers: history, class differences and clinical applicability. Curr Hypertens Rev. 2019;15(1):22–31. https://doi.org/10.2174/1573402114666180918102735.

21. Freund BJ, Joyner MJ, Jilka SM, et al. Thermoregulation during prolonged exercise in heat: alterations with beta-adrenergic blockade. J Appl Physiol. 1987;63(3):930–6. https://doi.org/10.1152/jappl.1987.63.3.930.

22. Abdelhafiz AH, Rodríguez-Mañas L, Morley JE, Sinclair AJ. Hypoglycemia in older people - a less well recognized risk factor for frailty. Aging Dis. 2015;6(2):156–67. https://doi.org/10.14336/ad.2014.0330.

23. Fonseca VA. Effects of beta-blockers on glucose and lipid metabolism. Curr Med Res Opin. 2010;26(3):615–29. https://doi.org/10.1185/03007990903533681.

24. Spranger MD, Krishnan AC, Levy PD, O'Leary DS, Smith SA. Blood flow restriction training and the exercise pressor reflex: a call for concern. Am J Physiol Heart Circ Physiol. 2015;309(9):1440–52. https://doi.org/10.1152/ajpheart.00208.2015.

25. Kleindorfer DO, Towfighi A, Chaturvedi S, et al. 2021 guideline for the prevention of stroke in patients with stroke and transient ischemic attack: a guideline from the American Heart Association/American Stroke Association. Stroke. 2021;52(7):e364–467. https://doi.org/10.1161/STR.0000000000000375.

26. Albaghdadi MS, Dudzinski DM, Giordano N, et al. Cardiopulmonary exercise testing in patients following massive and submassive pulmonary embolism. J Am Heart Assoc. 2018;7(5):e006841. https://doi.org/10.1161/jaha.117.006841.

27. Højen AA, Nielsen PB, Overvad TF, et al. Long-term management of pulmonary embolism: a review of consequences, treatment, and rehabilitation. J Clin Med. 2022;11(19):5970. https://doi.org/10.3390/jcm11195970.
28. Theis KA, Roblin DW, Helmick CG, Luo R, Prevalence and causes of work disability among working-age U.S. adults, 2011-2013, NHIS. Disabil Health J. 2018;11(1):108–15. https://doi.org/10.1016/j.dhjo.2017.04.010.
29. CDC. Arthritis related statistics. https://www.cdc.gov/arthritis/data_statistics/arthritis-related-stats.htm.
30. Arthritis Society C. The truth about arthritis. https://arthritis.ca/about-arthritis/what-is-arthritis/the-truth-about-arthritis.
31. American College of R. Exercise & Arthritis. https://rheumatology.org/exercise-and-arthritis.
32. England BR, Smith BJ, Baker NA, et al. 2022 American College of Rheumatology guideline for exercise, rehabilitation, diet, and additional integrative interventions for rheumatoid arthritis. Arthritis Care Res. 2023;75(8):1603–15. https://doi.org/10.1002/acr.25117.
33. Munneke M, de Jong Z, Zwinderman AH, et al. High intensity exercise or conventional exercise for patients with rheumatoid arthritis? Outcome expectations of patients, rheumatologists, and physiotherapists. Ann Rheum Dis. 2004;63(7):804–8. https://doi.org/10.1136/ard.2003.011189.
34. Maradit Kremers H, Larson DR, Crowson CS, et al. Prevalence of total hip and knee replacement in the United States. J Bone Joint Surg Am. 2015;97(17):1386–97. https://doi.org/10.2106/jbjs.N.01141.
35. Fortier LM, Rockov ZA, Chen AF, Rajaee SS. Activity recommendations after total hip and total knee arthroplasty. J Bone Joint Surg Am. 2021;103(5):446–55. https://doi.org/10.2106/jbjs.20.00983.
36. Kuster MS. Exercise recommendations after total joint replacement: a review of the current literature and proposal of scientifically based guidelines. Sports Med. 2002;32(7):433–45. https://doi.org/10.2165/00007256-200232070-00003.
37. van der Weegen W, Kornuijt A, Das D. Do lifestyle restrictions and precautions prevent dislocation after total hip arthroplasty? A systematic review and meta-analysis of the literature. Clin Rehabil. 2016;30(4):329–39. https://doi.org/10.1177/0269215515579421.
38. CDC. National Diabetes Statistics Report. https://www.cdc.gov/diabetes/data/statistics-report/index.html#print.
39. Colberg SR, Sigal RJ, Yardley JE, et al. Physical activity/exercise and diabetes: a position statement of the American Diabetes Association. Diabetes Care. 2016;39(11):2065–79. https://doi.org/10.2337/dc16-1728.
40. Kenny GP, Sigal RJ, McGinn R. Body temperature regulation in diabetes. Temperature. 2016;3(1):119–45. https://doi.org/10.1080/23328940.2015.1131506.
41. Kokkinos PF, Faselis C, Myers J, Panagiotakos D, Doumas M. Interactive effects of fitness and statin treatment on mortality risk in veterans with dyslipidaemia: a cohort study. Lancet. 2013;381(9864):394–9. https://doi.org/10.1016/s0140-6736(12)61426-3.
42. Selva-O'Callaghan A, Alvarado-Cardenas M, Pinal-Fernández I, et al. Statin-induced myalgia and myositis: an update on pathogenesis and clinical recommendations. Expert Rev Clin Immunol. 2018;14(3):215–24. https://doi.org/10.1080/1744666x.2018.1440206.
43. Gupta A, Thompson D, Whitehouse A, et al. Adverse events associated with unblinded, but not with blinded, statin therapy in the Anglo-Scandinavian Cardiac Outcomes Trial-Lipid-Lowering Arm (ASCOT-LLA): a randomised double-blind placebo-controlled trial and its non-randomised non-blind extension phase. Lancet. 2017;389(10088):2473–81. https://doi.org/10.1016/s0140-6736(17)31075-9.
44. Wilund KR, Viana JL, Perez LM. A critical review of exercise training in hemodialysis patients: personalized activity prescriptions are needed. Exerc Sport Sci Rev. 2020;48(1):28–39. https://doi.org/10.1249/jes.0000000000000209.

45. Johansen KL. Exercise and dialysis. Hemodial Int. 2008;12(3):290–300. https://doi.org/10.1111/j.1542-4758.2008.00269.x.
46. Davenport A. Why is intradialytic hypotension the commonest complication of outpatient dialysis treatments? Kidney Int Rep. 2023;8(3):405–18. https://doi.org/10.1016/j.ekir.2022.10.031.
47. NIDDK. Peritoneal dialysis.
48. Spruit MA, Burtin C, De Boever P, et al. COPD and exercise: does it make a difference? Breathe. 2016;12(2):38–49. https://doi.org/10.1183/20734735.003916.
49. American Lung A. Physical activity and COPD. https://www.lung.org/lung-health-diseases/lung-disease-lookup/copd/living-with-copd/physical-activity#:~:text=Exercising%20for%20too%20long%20or,or%20other%20COPD%20related%20symptoms.
50. Cleveland C. COPD: Exercise precautions. https://my.clevelandclinic.org/health/articles/9448-copd-exercise-precautions.
51. Boriek AM, Lopez MA, Velasco C, et al. Obesity modulates diaphragm curvature in subjects with and without COPD. Am J Physiol Regul Integr Comp Physiol. 2017;313(5):620–9. https://doi.org/10.1152/ajpregu.00173.2017.
52. Goh JT, Balmain BN, Wilhite DP, et al. Elevated risk of dyspnea in adults with obesity. Respir Physiol Neurobiol. 2023;318:104151. https://doi.org/10.1016/j.resp.2023.104151.
53. Eves ND, Davidson WJ. Evidence-based risk assessment and recommendations for physical activity clearance: respiratory disease. Appl Physiol Nutr Metab. 2011;36(1):80–100. https://doi.org/10.1139/h11-057.
54. Eichenberger PA, Diener SN, Kofmehl R, Spengler CM. Effects of exercise training on airway hyperreactivity in asthma: a systematic review and meta-analysis. Sports Med. 2013;43(11):1157–70. https://doi.org/10.1007/s40279-013-0077-2.
55. American Lung A. Being active with asthma. https://www.lung.org/lung-health-diseases/lung-disease-lookup/asthma/managing-asthma/asthma-and-exercise.
56. Mayo C. Exercise-induced asthma. https://www.mayoclinic.org/diseases-conditions/exercise-induced-asthma/symptoms-causes/syc-20372300.
57. Schmitz KH, Courneya KS, Matthews C, et al. American College of Sports Medicine roundtable on exercise guidelines for cancer survivors. Med Sci Sports Exerc. 2010;42(7):1409–26. https://doi.org/10.1249/MSS.0b013e3181e0c112.
58. American College of Sports M. Moving through cancer. https://www.exerciseismedicine.org/eim-in-action/moving-through-cancer-2/.
59. Yu JT, Xu W, Tan CC, et al. Evidence-based prevention of Alzheimer's disease: systematic review and meta-analysis of 243 observational prospective studies and 153 randomised controlled trials. J Neurol Neurosurg Psychiatry. 2020;91(11):1201–9. https://doi.org/10.1136/jnnp-2019-321913.
60. Iso-Markku P, Kujala UM, Knittle K, Polet J, Vuoksimaa E, Waller K. Physical activity as a protective factor for dementia and Alzheimer's disease: systematic review, meta-analysis and quality assessment of cohort and case-control studies. Br J Sports Med. 2022;56(12):701–9. https://doi.org/10.1136/bjsports-2021-104981.
61. Alzheimer's S. Physical exercise and dementia. https://www.alzheimers.org.uk/about-dementia/risk-factors-and-prevention/physical-exercise.
62. National Institute on A. Staying physically active with Alzheimer's. https://www.nia.nih.gov/health/staying-physically-active-alzheimers#:~:text=Being%20active%20and%20getting%20exercise,and%20heart%20in%20good%20shape.
63. Alzheimer's A. 24/7 wandering support for a safe return. https://www.alz.org/help-support/caregiving/safety/medicalert-with-24-7-wandering-support.
64. Burfield M, Sayers M, Buhmann R. The association between running volume and knee osteoarthritis prevalence: a systematic review and meta-analysis. Phys Ther Sport. 2023;61:1–10. https://doi.org/10.1016/j.ptsp.2023.02.003.
65. Dhillon J, Kraeutler MJ, Belk JW, et al. Effects of running on the development of knee osteoarthritis: an updated systematic review at short-term follow-up. Orthop J Sports Med. 2023;11(3):23259671231152900. https://doi.org/10.1177/23259671231152900.

Resources

National Senior Games Association.

Rikli RE, Jones CJ. Senior fitness test manual. 2nd ed. Champaign: Human Kinetics; 2013.

Thompson PD, Baggish AL, Franklin B, Jaworski C, Riebe D. American College of Sports Medicine expert consensus statement to update recommendations for screening, staffing, and emergency policies to prevent cardiovascular events at health fitness facilities. Curr Sports Med Rep. 2020;19(6):223–31.

U.S. Department of Health and Human Services. Physical activity guidelines for Americans. 2nd ed. Washington: U.S. Department of Health and Human Services; 2018.

Chapter 4
Types of Exercise: Flexibility, Strengthening, Endurance, Balance

Lynn B. Panton and Ashley L. Artese

Key Points

- Key components of a well-rounded exercise program are flexibility, strength, endurance, and balance training, but older adults may prefer or need to start with one or two components
- Flexibility training requires stretches to maintain or improve range of motion around joints, prevent injury, and reduce joint pain
- Strength or resistance training engages various muscle groups using weights, resistance bands, or other methods to improve muscle strength, bone density, and lean muscle mass
- Endurance or aerobic training involves sustained movement of large muscle groups to elevate the heart rate, with benefits for cardiovascular fitness and many health conditions
- A general rule of thumb for determining starting levels for exercise components is "start low, go slow": start at low intensities and progress gradually

Supplementary Information The online version contains supplementary material available at https://doi.org/10.1007/978-3-031-52928-3_4.

L. B. Panton (✉)
Florida State University, Tallahassee, FL, USA
e-mail: lpanton@fsu.edu

A. L. Artese
Department of Exercise Science and Health Promotion, Florida Atlantic University, Boca Raton, FL, USA
e-mail: aartese@fau.edu

Introduction

A well-rounded exercise program consists of flexibility, strength, endurance, and balance training. These four components are essential for the promotion of healthy aging and the maintenance of functional capacity, mobility, independence, and quality of life [1–3]. *Flexibility training* can help maintain or improve range of motion around joints, which may prevent injury, reduce joint pain, and improve posture. This component may consist of dynamic stretches that involve actively moving through the joint's range of motion or static stretches that are held for a certain length of time. *Strength training,* also known as weight or resistance training, requires the contraction of a muscle against a weight or type of resistance to build or maintain the strength and endurance of the muscle. It can be achieved using machines, free weights, resistance bands, body weight, or water resistance. Strength training is important for maintaining or improving muscle strength, lean muscle mass, and bone density, which allows older adults to better perform activities of daily living. *Endurance training*, also known as aerobic training, involves the continuous movement of major muscle groups such as the legs or arms, to maintain an elevated heart rate for an extended period of time. Modes of endurance exercise may include walking, cycling, stair climbing, dancing, or swimming. Endurance training equipment such as treadmills, cycle ergometers, ellipticals, stair steppers, and rowing machines can also be used. Endurance training helps to maintain the health of the heart and lungs, aids in the prevention of many chronic diseases such as heart disease and diabetes, and can reduce the risk and severity of infections and illnesses. Since the risk of falling increases with age, *balance training* serves as an important activity for fall prevention. It involves exercises that are designed to challenge an individual's ability to stabilize his or her body and maintain posture through the use of unstable surfaces, narrowing bases of support, weight shifts, or the removal of upper body assistance.

Healthy older adults do not need a health screening prior to starting a moderate-intensity exercise program, such as walking or an older adult exercise class (see Chap. 3). Older adults with chronic medical conditions should be assessed by a clinician to identify health risks or safety concerns. Although being sedentary is more detrimental to the older adult's health than participating in a moderate-intensity exercise program [4], the clinician should determine whether an exercise program needs to be adjusted for the older adult's chronic conditions, medications, and current functional level. A baseline physical assessment is valuable to evaluate the older adult's fitness and functional abilities in order to determine an appropriate starting point for the exercise program. Physical assessments such as the Senior Fitness Test, Short Physical Performance Battery, and National Institute of Aging Tool Kit may be used to assess fitness levels for flexibility, strength, endurance, and balance depending on the older adult's physical capability for performing these tests [5, 6]. In addition, questionnaires relating to lifestyle, physical activity, fears, and physical activity readiness [4] are helpful to assess the older adult's current physical activity levels as well as identify additional risks, barriers, apprehensions, and views toward exercise. Once these assessments are completed, a suitable plan of action can be determined (for more information on writing an exercise prescription, see Chap. 6).

When planning an exercise program for an older adult, it is important for safety and adherence to begin slowly at low intensities and gradually progress from there. While a well-rounded program should consist of the four components, starting an older adult with a program that consists of flexibility, strength, endurance, and balance exercises may be overwhelming. Therefore, it may be more beneficial, especially in those who are sedentary or have functional limitations, to begin with one or two components (e.g., flexibility, strength) and slowly incorporate additional ones as the older adult progresses [3]. For older adults who are already active and have a higher level of fitness, a moderate-intensity program consisting of two or more fitness components, suitable for their fitness level and goals, may be prescribed. For those with impaired function or who are bedridden, flexibility should be incorporated first to increase range of motion and decrease stiffness in the joints. Eventually strength training can be integrated, with exercises and resistances that are appropriate for the older adult's fitness level and health condition. This may include exercises performed while lying down, seated in a chair, standing, in the pool, or using resistance machines. If the older adult cannot support his or her body weight independently, the initial components should be strength and balance training, before moving to walking and other forms of weight bearing endurance activity. As strength and fitness levels progress, a form of endurance exercise may then be added followed by additional balance training to provide a comprehensive exercise program promoting fitness, independence, and healthy aging for the older adult [3].

Flexibility Training

Flexibility training allows older adults to maintain or improve their ability to perform activities of daily living, such as combing hair, reaching for objects on a shelf or the floor, getting dressed, or putting on shoes. Flexibility training, especially exercises focusing on the hip extensors, also improves several gait parameters, such as speed, stride length, and cadence, which may result in increased mobility and reduced risk for falling [7]. In addition, stretching can help prevent injuries such as muscle strains or pulls as well as reduce pain in areas such as the knee, hip, lower back, and neck.

For improvements in flexibility, the American College of Sports Medicine (ACSM) recommends performing static stretches for all major muscle groups at least 2 days/week. Each stretch should be held without bouncing for 30–60 s and repeated 3–4 times [4]. Static flexibility exercises should be performed after endurance or

Table 4.1 Important instructions and safety cues for stretching

• Stretch after endurance or strength exercises or make sure muscles are properly warmed up before stretching to avoid injury
• Gradually move into the stretch. Avoid bouncing movements
• Stretches should be held in a position where mild discomfort is felt, but never pain
• Maintain slow and steady breathing; be sure to exhale when moving into the stretch
• Some stretches may require the older adult to lie down or take a seat on the floor. If he or she has a fear of getting on the floor or does not have the strength to stand back up, suggest a seated or standing stretch for the same muscle group or encourage the use of a couch or bed. Make sure that the surface is large enough to avoid a fall

strength training to ensure that muscles are warm. This enables older adults to gain the most benefit from the stretches and reduces the risk for injury. For weak or bedridden patients who are starting out with only flexibility training, it is important to instruct those individuals to gradually move the muscle through its range of motion, for a slow dynamic movement, or gently move into and hold the static stretch. Flexibility exercises can be performed while lying down, seated, or standing using props such as a chair, wall, or band for assistance if needed (see Table 4.1).

Flexibility Exercises

Pictures and descriptions of each exercise are presented below. Start the individual off slowly by choosing 2–4 stretches for the lower body and 4–6 stretches for the upper body to target all major muscle groups.

Lower Body Stretches
Supine hamstrings stretch (see Fig. 4.1)

Supine Hamstrings Stretch

1. Lie down with the lower back pressed into the floor, kness bent at a 90° angle, and feet flat on the floor.
2. Extend the right leg towards the ceiling. Place the hands behind the thigh, calf, or ankle and gently pull the leg towards the body until the stretch is felt in the hamstrings.
3. Flex the foot to increase the stretch in the hamstrings and calf muscles.
4. Repeat on the other side.

   Modifications/Props:
   1. Place a band or towel near the ball of the foot and gently pull the leg forward with the band until the stretch is felt.
   2. Place extended leg against the wall (heel rested on the wall) and hold.

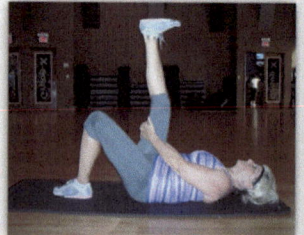

Fig. 4.1 Lower body stretches. Supine hamstrings stretch

Seated hamstrings stretch (see Fig. 4.2)

Seated Hamstrings Stretch

1. Start seated on the floor or bed with both legs extended with heels touching the floor and feet flexed.
2. Bend the left knee and place the sole of the foot against the right inner thigh.
3. Square the shoulders to the extended leg and exhale while moving forward at the hips, reaching both hands toward the right ankle or foot.
4. Repeat on the other side.

   Modifications/Props:
   - For those with extremely tight hamstrings, the hips can be elevated by sitting on a pillow or folded blanket while performing this stretch.
   - Place a band around the extended foot and gently pull the upper body forward.

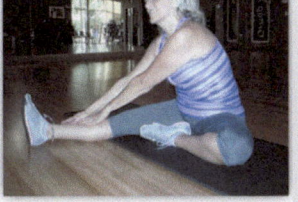

Fig. 4.2 Lower body stretches. Seated hamstrings stretch

Chair Hamstrings Stretch

1. Start seated in a chair with knees bent at a 90° angle and both feet placed flat on the floor.
2. Extend the right leg straight and place the right heel on the floor.
3. Slowly hinge forward at the hips, reaching both hands equally towards the right foot.
4. Repeat on the other side.

   Modifications/Props
   - For those who may feel pain in the lower back when leaning forward, this exercise can be modified to maintain back support against the chair. Place a band or a towel under the foot of the extended leg and gently pull on the band to lift the right leg off the floor for the stretch.

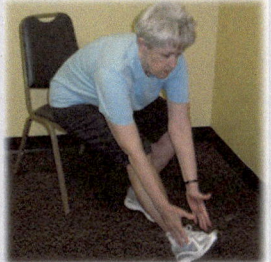

Fig. 4.3 Lower body stretches. Chair hamstrings stretch

Standing Quadriceps Stretch

1. Stand with feet flat on the floor and knees slightly bent. Place hand on a chair or the wall for support.
2. Bend the right knee and lift the right heel towards the left gluteal muscles.
3. Reach the left hand behind the body and take hold of the right ankle.
4. Keep knees next to each other with the bent knee pointing down towards the floor, not out to the side.
5. Repeat on the other side.

   Modifications/Props:
   - If the patient has difficulty holding the ankle, the elevated foot can be placed on a chair instead.

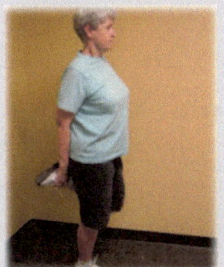

Fig. 4.4 Lower body stretches. Standing quadriceps stretch

Chair hamstrings stretch (see Fig. 4.3)
Standing quadriceps stretch (see Fig. 4.4)
Standing calf stretch (see Fig. 4.5)

Supine hip rotator stretch (see Fig. 4.6)

Standing Calf Stretch

1. Stand facing a wall with feet about hip or shoulder-width apart, and place the hands against the wall at about eye level.
2. Place the right leg one or two feet behind the left leg.
3. Draw both heels down towards the floor and slowly bend the front knee until a stretch is felt in the right calf muscles. Do not let the front knee pass the toes.
4. Repeat on the other side.

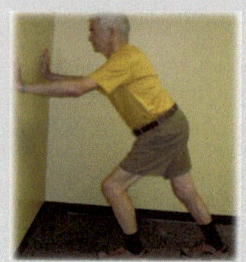

Fig. 4.5 Lower body stretches. Standing calf stretch

Chair hip rotator stretch (see Fig. 4.7)

Supine Hip Rotator Stretch

1. Start out lying with the lower back pressed into the floor, knees bent at a 90° angle, and feet flat on the floor.
2. Place the right ankle on the left thigh near the left knee.
3. Gently push on the right leg to open the hip until you feel a stretch in the right hip and thigh.
4. Repeat on the other side.

   Modifications/Props:
   - To further stretch the gluteal muscles: with the right ankle crossed over the left thigh, reach the hands between the legs and take hold of the left thigh. Slowly pull the left knee towards the chest to feel a stretch in the right gluteal muscles.

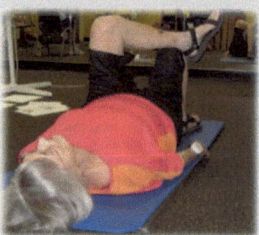

Fig. 4.6 Lower body stretches. Supine hip rotator stretch

Seated gluteal stretch (see Fig. 4.8)

Chair Hip Rotator Stretch

1. Start out seated in a chair with knees bent at a 90° angle and both feet flat on the floor.
2. Bend the right knee and place the right ankle on the left thigh near the left knee.
3. Gently push the right thigh and knee towards the floor until a stretch is felt in the right hip and thigh.
4. Repeat on the other side.

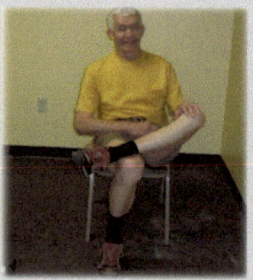

Fig. 4.7 Lower body stretches. Chair hip rotator stretch

Seated butterfly groin stretch (see Fig. 4.9)

Seated Gluteal Stretch

1. Start out seated on the floor or bed with legs extended.
2. Bend the right knee and place the right foot on the outside of the left thigh.
3. Slowly start to twist the upper body to the right side, keeping the upper body upright.
4. The left arm can wrap around the right leg or push against the outside of the right leg for a deeper stretch.
5. Repeat on the other side.

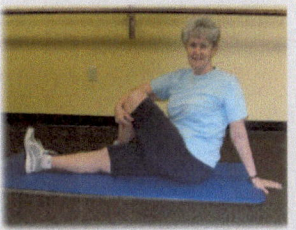

Fig. 4.8 Lower body stretches. Seated gluteal stretch

Standing groin stretch (see Fig. 4.10)

Seated Butterfly Groin Stretch

1. Sit on the floor with the back straight, shoulders down, abdominals tight, soles of the feet together in front of body, and knees bent to the sides.
2. Pull heel towards body while simultaneously relaxing the knees towards the floor.

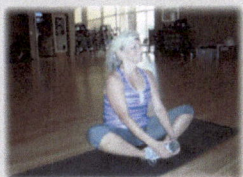

Fig. 4.9 Lower body stretches. Seated butterfly groin stretch

Standing Groin Stretch

1. Start in a standing position with hands on hips or upper thighs.
2. Lean to the side and bend the right knee while keeping the left leg straight.
3. Press the hips back as you lunge and keep both feet pointing forward.
4. Hold and then repeat on the opposite side.

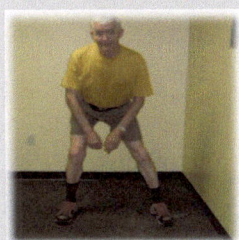

Fig. 4.10 Lower body stretches. Standing groin stretch

Upper Body Stretches

Chest and biceps stretch (see Fig. 4.11)

Chest and Biceps Stretch

1. Stand or sit up tall and place the arms behind the back with thumbs facing down. Clasp hands together if possible.
2. Once the arms are extended behind, gently pull arms upward until a stretch is felt in the chest and biceps.

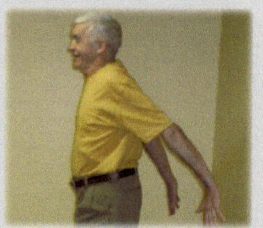

Fig. 4.11 Upper body stretches. Chest and biceps stretch

Triceps stretch (see Fig. 4.12)
Shoulder stretch (see Fig. 4.13)

Triceps Stretch

1. Lift both arms above the head and bend elbows so that forearms are behind the head (but not resting on it).
2. Try to point the right elbow to the sky.
3. Gently grasp the left elbow with the right hand.
4. Allow the left hand to drop towards the middle of the shoulder blades.
5. Feel the stretch on the outside of the upper left arm.
6. Gently pull the left elbow towards the right shoulder to deepen the stretch.
7. Repeat with opposite arm.

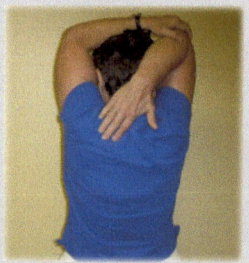

Fig. 4.12 Upper body stretches. Triceps stretch

Neck stretch (see Fig. 4.14)
Upper back stretch (see Fig. 4.15)

Shoulder Stretch

1. Start in a seated or standing position.
2. Place the right arm across the chest.
3. Support the right arm by placing the left hand against the right forearm to feel a stretch in the right shoulder.
4. Repeat on the other side.

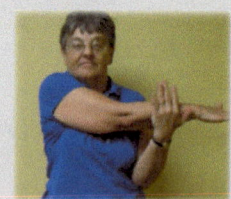

Fig. 4.13 Upper body stretches. Shoulder stretch

Supine lower back stretch (see Fig. 4.16)

Neck Stretch

1. Start in a seated or standing position.
2. Slowly lower the chin towards the chest until a stretch is felt in the muscles in the back of the neck.
3. Return to starting position and then lower the right ear towards the right shoulder and hold.
4. Repeat on the other side.

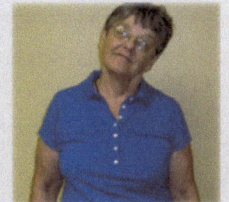

Fig. 4.14 Upper body stretches. Neck stretch

Seated lower back stretch (see Fig. 4.17)

Upper Back Stretch

1. Start in a seated or standing position.
2. Extend the arms out in front.
3. Place one hand in front of the other with the palms facing towards or away from the body.
4. Press both hands away from the body, allowing the upper back to be slightly rounded.

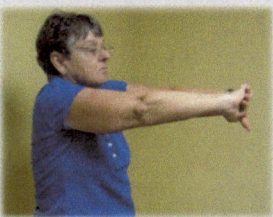

Fig. 4.15 Upper body stretches. Upper back stretch

Abdominal stretch (see Fig. 4.18)

Supine Lower Back Stretch

1. Start out lying on the floor with the lower back pressed into the floor.
2. Bend the knees and slowly draw the knees toward the chest by reaching the hands behind the hamstrings.

   *Modifications/Props:
   * This can be done by pulling one knee at a time towards the chest.

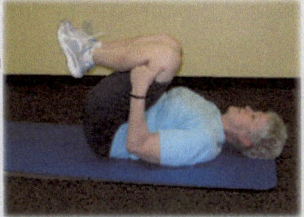

Fig. 4.16 (Lower back/abdominal stretches. Supine lower back stretch

Seated Lower Back Stretch

1. Start out seated in a sturdy chair that has four legs (Do not use a rocking chair or recliner)
2. Slowly lean forward and allow the arms to move towards the floor.

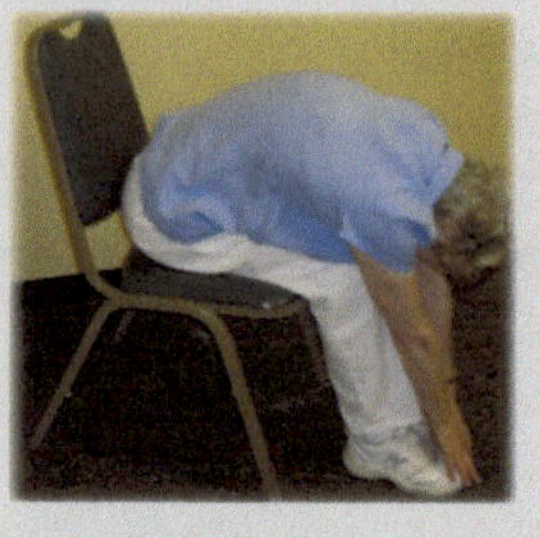

Fig. 4.17 Lower back/abdominal stretches. Seated lower back stretch

Abdominal Stretch

1. Start out lying face down on the floor or bed.
2. Place the forearms on the floor with the elbows directly underneath the shoulders.
3. Slowly push the upper body up off of the mat and hold.

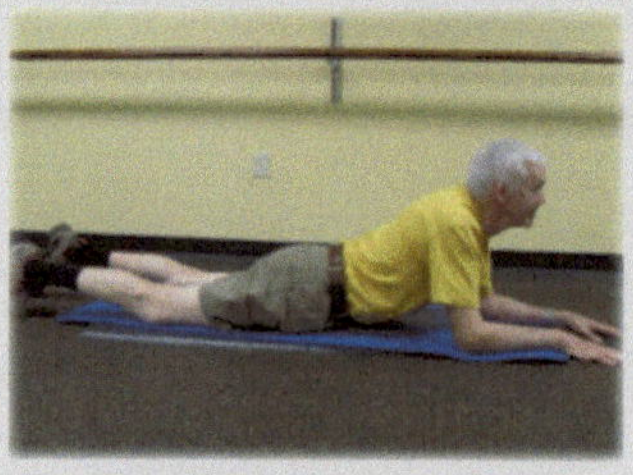

Fig. 4.18 Lower back/abdominal stretches. Abdominal stretch

Strength Training

Older adults who regularly participate in a strength training program will maintain or improve muscular strength and function, bone density, and body composition as well as reduce fall risk [8]. Strength training can also address symptoms of many conditions including arthritis, osteoporosis, diabetes, and depression [8]. It is recommended by ACSM that older adults participate in strength training activities for 2–3 days/week [4]. Start out slowly with a program consisting of 10–14 exercises that target all major muscle groups. Each exercise should be completed for one set of 10–15 repetitions. A set refers to a group or round of repetitions completed at one time. Over time, the number of sets for each exercise can be gradually increased to 2 or 3. Exercises can be prescribed using a variety of equipment such as machines, free weights, resistance bands, and stability balls. Fancy equipment does not have to be purchased. Milk jugs filled with water or sand, soup cans, or books can also be used for resistance. Body weight exercises can also be used. For those individuals who are bedridden or confined to a chair, exercises can be performed while lying down or seated. For those who have more mobility, it may be beneficial to start off with machines to provide support when learning new exercises and to promote

Table 4.2 Important instructions and safety cues for strength training

• When seated in a machine or chair or lying down on a mat, the small of the back should be pressed firmly against the seat or mat surface
• When seated, make sure knees are bent at a 90° angle with feet flat on the floor
• Perform movements slowly, and allow 2–3 s for the lifting phase and 3–4 s for the lowering phase
• Always breathe. Never hold the breath—exhale during the lifting phase and inhale during the lowering phase
• Be sure to gently hold the weight. Avoid squeezing or tightly gripping weights
• Make sure the neck and spine are aligned when lifting
• For older adults with balance issues, all exercises should be completed while seated in a chair or lying on a firm surface. As the older adult becomes stronger and balance improves, the older adult can move from a supine to sitting to standing position, for strength training exercises

safety and proper lifting technique. Once the older adult feels comfortable with machines, more functional movements can be incorporated into the training program to promote balance, use of stabilizing muscles, and multi-joint movements. Functional movements are those that are more specific to everyday activities, such as bending down or lifting an object to place on a shelf. For frail individuals, doing functional movements that simulate daily activities should be included, such as sit-to-stand exercises from a chair or step ups (see Table 4.2).

Strength Exercises

Strength exercises may be performed at home or in a fitness facility. If it is determined that the older adult's program will include resistance machines, follow the safety and usage directions provided by the manufacturing company for each machine. Regardless of the mode of strength training, start an older adult slowly with 4–6 exercises for the lower body and 6–8 exercises for the upper body, lower back, and abdominal muscles to target all major muscle groups. If ten exercises are too much for the older adult, choose one or two exercises each for the upper and lower body. Then slowly increase the number of exercises over time. For example, if the older adult is struggling to get out of a chair, doing an exercise that incorporates the gluteal muscles and the arms (triceps) could be completed in the first few weeks before additional exercises are added. Begin with one set of 10–15 repetitions at an intensity level of 65–75% of one repetition maximum (1RM), which is equivalent to the amount of weight that can be lifted for a maximum of 10–15 repetitions. Encourage the older adult to perform the strength program for a minimum of 2–3 days/week, while allowing at least 1 day of rest between exercise sessions. Gradually progress every 3–4 weeks by modifying one of the following: frequency, intensity, repetitions, or set number. In addition, each exercise can be replaced with a more challenging intensity option or a new exercise. Before strength training, the older adult needs to warm up with exercises that increase blood flow and body temperature such as slow walking, cycling, or marching in place.

Upper Body Strength Training Exercises
Chest press (see Fig. 4.19)

Chest Press

1. Start out lying with the lower back pressed into the mat, knees bent at a 90° angle, and feet flat on the floor.
2. Hold a weight in each hand and extend the arms out to the side so that elbows are in line with the chest and bent at a 90° angle.
3. Exhale and slowly extend the arms to press the weights forward until the weights meet above the chest.
4. Inhale and return to starting position.

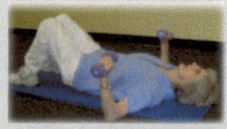
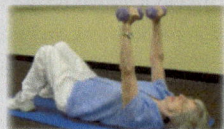

Fig. 4.19 Upper body strength training exercises. Chest press

Upright row (see Fig. 4.20)

Upright Row

1. Start out standing with feet hip-width apart, holding a weight in each hand.
2. Extend the arms straight so that the weights are in front of the thighs with the palms facing towards the leg.
3. Exhale and slowly lift the weights towards the chest by bending the elbows out to the sides.
4. Hold for a second when the weights reach the chest and then inhale as weights are returned to starting position.

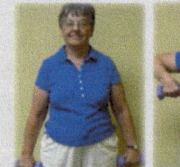
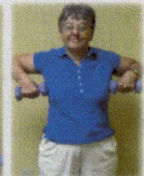

Fig. 4.20 Upper body strength training exercises. Upright row

Front shoulder raises (see Fig. 4.21)

Front Shoulder Raise

1. Start out standing or seated in a chair with the back supported and feet flat on the floor.
2. Hold a weight in each hand with arms by the sides with the palms facing back.
3. Exhale and slowly raise the arms out to the front, keeping the elbow extended and the palms facing down.
4. Stop when the arms reach shoulder level and then slowly lower the weights back down.

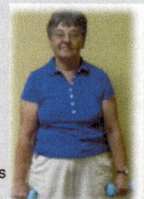
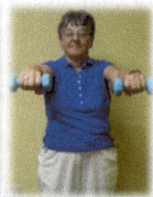

Fig. 4.21 Upper body strength training exercises. Front shoulder raises

Biceps curl (see Fig. 4.22)

Biceps Curl

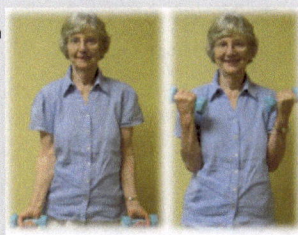

1. Start standing or seated in a chair with the back supported and feet flat on the floor.
2. Hold a weight in each hand and extend the arms straight by the sides of the body,palms facing forward.
3. With the elbows pressed firmly against the side, exhale and slowly bend\ the elbows, bringing the forearms closer to the upper arms.
4. Hold for a second and then inhale to return to starting position.

Fig. 4.22   Upper body strength training exercises. Biceps curl

Standing triceps extension (see Fig. 4.23)

Standing Triceps Extension

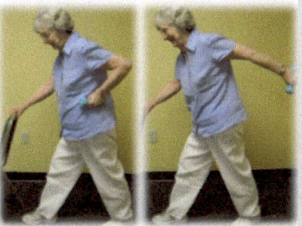

1. Start out standing behind a chair with one foot in front of the other. Slowly bend forward at the hips to about a 45° angle and place the left hand on the chair for support.
2. Hold a weight in the right hand and bend the elbow, sending it back behind the body with the right arm close to the side of the body.
3. Slowly extend the elbow, bringing the weight behind the body while exhaling.
4. Hold for a second, and then return to starting position.

Fig. 4.23   Upper body strength training exercises. Standing triceps extension

Lower Body Strength Training Exercises
Seated leg extensions (see Fig. 4.24)

Seated Leg Extensions

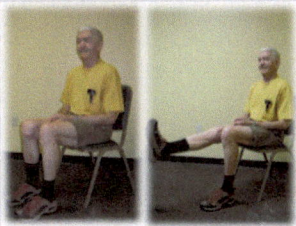

1. Start seated in a chair with the back supported and feet flat on the floor.
2. Exhale and slowly lift the right foot off the floor and extend the right leg out in front, making sure the right knee stays slightly bent on the extension.
3. Hold for one second. Inhale and return to starting position.
4. Repeat for the desired amount of repetitions before switching to the other leg.
5. Ankle weights can be added for increased resistance.

Fig. 4.24   Lower body strength training exercises. Seated leg extensions

Standing hamstrings curl (see Fig. 4.25)

Standing Hamstrings Curl

1. Stand behind a chair with feet flat on the floor, shoulder-width apart.
2. Slowly shift the weight onto the left leg. Exhale and flex the right knee to lift the right heel up towards the gluteal muscles. Hold when the knee reaches a 90° bend.
3. Inhale and slowly return to starting position.
4. Repeat for the desired amount of repetitions before switching to the other leg.
5. Ankle weights can be added for increased resistance.

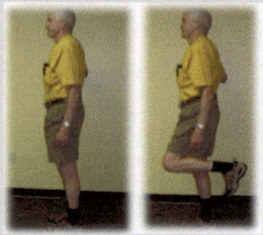

Fig. 4.25 Lower body strength training exercises. Standing hamstrings curl

Standing calf raises (see Fig. 4.26)

Standing Calf Raises

1. Stand behind a chair or near the wall with feet hip-width apart and both hands holding onto the back of the chair or wall for support.
2. Exhale and slowly raise the heels off of the floor, being sure to maintain an upright body position.
3. Inhale and lower the heels back to the floor. Repeat for desired amount of repetitions.
4. Ankle weights can be added to increase resistance.

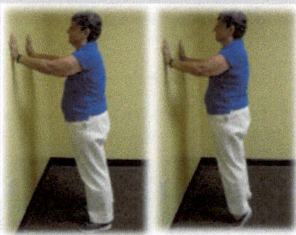

Fig. 4.26 Lower body strength training exercises. Standing calf raises

Chair Squats

1. Start seated in the middle of a chair with legs about hip-width apart and feet flat on the floor placed about 5-8 inches in front of the chair.
2. Arms can be extended out in front, crossed over the chest, or placed on the chair handles if arm assistance is needed for the exercise.
3. Slowly exhale and stand up, making sure the knees do not fully extend at the top of the movement.
4. Once reaching a full standing position, inhale and slowly lower the body down to a seated position on the chair, making sure not to allow knees to come past toes during the movement.
5. Hold for a second and repeat.

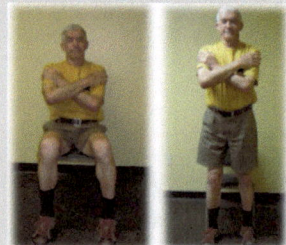

Fig. 4.27 Lower body strength training exercises. Chair squats

Chair squats (see Fig. 4.27)

Supine hip lifts (see Fig. 4.28)

Supine Hip Lifts

1. Lie on the back with arms by the sides and palms facing down. Knees should be bent at a 90° angle with feet flat on the floor.
2. Exhale and slowly raise the pelvis off the floor so that the lower back and buttoks are lifted.
3. Hold this position for 1-2 seconds.
4. Inhale and return to starting position and repeat.

   Modifications/Props:
   - To increase difficulty, this exercise can be performed on a single leg with the other leg lifted.

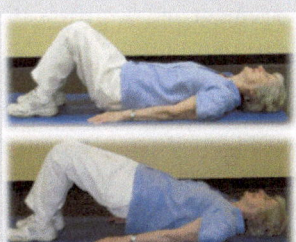

Fig. 4.28 Lower body strength training exercises. Supine hip lifts

Lower Back/Abdominal Exercises

Abdominal crunch (see Fig. 4.29)

Abdominal Crunch

1. Lie on the back with feet flat and knees bent. Make sure the small of the back is placed firmly against the mat.
2. Place the hands behind the head for support and slowly lift the head and shoulders off the floor, exhaling while contracting the abdominal muscles. Be sure to keep some space between the chin and the chest.
3. Try to imagine a string attached to the middle of chest (the sternum) pulling the upper body towards the ceiling without altering the head and neck position.
4. Hold for one second and then slowly return to starting position while inhaling.

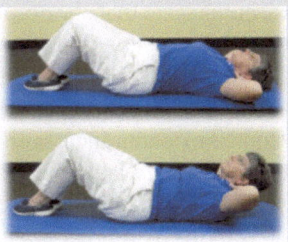

Fig. 4.29 Lower back/abdominal exercises. Abdominal crunch

Back Extensions

1. Lie face down with the hands under the chin or by the sides of the body.
2. Exhale and slowly lift the shoulders and chest off of the floor, keeping the neck in a neutral position.
3. Hold for 1-2 seconds and then slowly return to starting position.

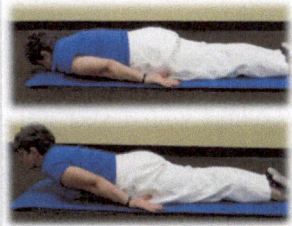

Fig. 4.30 Lower back/abdominal exercises. Back extensions

Back extensions (see Fig. 4.30)

Endurance Training

Endurance training, also known as aerobic or cardio training, is crucial for improving the function of the heart, lungs, and vascular system. It also aids in weight management and decreases the risk of chronic diseases such as cardiovascular disease, chronic obstructive pulmonary disease (COPD), type 2 diabetes, hypertension, arthritis, and dementia. Individuals who are more fit may have a stronger immune system, which can reduce the risk of contracting infectious diseases or the severity of symptoms from infectious diseases, including COVID-19 [9]. In addition, older adults with increased cardiovascular fitness can perform more difficult physical tasks and exercise at higher intensities than those who do not partake in regular endurance activities. It is recommended that adults ages 65 years and older accumulate a minimum of 150 min of moderate-intensity aerobic activity or 75 min of vigorous-intensity activity per week [4]. Moderate intensity can be identified as an intensity that causes the individual to be slightly out of breath or break a sweat, but still can carry on a conversation while exercising. Both the intensity and the recommended duration may seem strenuous and perhaps difficult to achieve for an older adult who is just starting an exercise program. Therefore, it is important to encourage the older adult to start out slowly with low-impact exercises such as walking outdoors or on a treadmill for a short duration, and gradually progress from there. Also, emphasize that shorter bouts of endurance exercise can be completed throughout the day to accumulate a total of 30 min/day.

Endurance exercise is generally associated with the use of equipment such as treadmills, elliptical machines, stair climbers, or a stationary cycle. However, a great advantage of endurance exercise is that it does not have to involve equipment and can be performed anywhere, at any time. Encourage the older adult to start with an activity in which he or she feels comfortable doing and to choose something enjoyable. Walking is a great way to start, but other options may include line dancing, group exercise classes, swimming, water-based exercise, or simple aerobic exercise moves at home. Walking is probably the easiest form of endurance training to do since special skills are not needed. An older adult can walk anywhere (inside or outside) without special equipment except a good pair of shoes. In addition, a portion of the recommended 150 min of exercise per week can be achieved by incorporating more active lifestyle habits, such as gardening, cleaning, taking the stairs instead of the elevator, or parking the car further away from a building entrance. For older adults with severe arthritis, peripheral neuropathy, neuromuscular disease, orthostatic hypotension, or balance/mobility issues, activities such as water aerobics, seated steppers, or recumbent cycles may be better alternatives to weight bearing exercises. Arm ergometry may also be a modality for endurance training for individuals who have had a stroke, amputation, leg ulcers or other conditions that

Table 4.3 Starting an endurance exercise program

• Start out slowly with a mode of endurance exercise. Slowly progress by increasing the time, intensity, or step count (measured by an activity monitor) by 10% every 1–2 weeks
• Monitor intensity with a rate of perceived exertion (RPE) scale (Table 4.4). On a scale of 1–10, moderate activity should feel like a 5 or 6. The RPE Scale can also be used to measure intensity when heart rate cannot be used due to arrhythmias, beta-blocker medications, or pacemakers [3]
• Measure progress using an activity tracker (watch, pedometer, or cell phone), which can track the number of steps taken. By setting weekly step goals, the older adult can be motivated to increase total daily steps, with the ultimate target being 10,000 steps/day for healthy older adults
• Wear shoes that offer support and are appropriate for the type of activity

Table 4.4 Rating of perceived exertion scale

Rating of perceived exertion (RPE) scale	
10	Maximal
9	Extremely hard
8	Really hard
7	
6	Hard
5	Challenging
4	Moderate
3	Easy
2	Really easy
1	Rest

would make lower limb training difficult. Again, with individuals who are frail, introducing flexibility and low level strength training first, followed by balance training and finally endurance training is recommended (see Tables 4.3 and 4.4).

Endurance Exercises

A variety of endurance exercises or sequences can be performed at a fitness facility, pool, or at home. Endurance exercise involves the elevation of the heart rate for a sustained period of time. These exercises are meant to be continued for an allotted amount of time. The older adult may decide to walk, or he or she may combine the endurance exercises listed below to add more variety and multi-directional movements into the workout.

Land Exercises

Walking

1. Walk with body erect, head lifted, and shoulders relaxed.
2. Let the arms swing naturally at the sides of the body.
3. When taking a step, place the heel on the floor first, and roll through to the ball of the foot.
4. Walk at a comfortable pace that allows conversation, but with increased rate of breathing.

Side Steps

1. Start in a standing position with feet together.
2. Step the right foot out to the side about 2–3 feet, being sure to keep the toes always facing forward.
3. Step the left foot in to meet the right foot so that feet are now together.
4. Step the left foot out to the left side, and then step the right foot in to return to starting position.
5. Let the arms move in and out naturally with each step. Repeat.

Heel Digs

1. Start in a standing position with feet together and the arms bent with elbows by the sides of the body.
2. Lift the right leg and place the right heel on the floor in front while extending the elbows, pressing the hands toward the floor.
3. Place the right foot back on the floor and repeat the movement with the left foot.

High Knees

1. Start out standing with feet flat on the floor.
2. Slowly lift the right foot off the floor, lifting the knee at a comfortable height. Do not let the hip flex beyond a 90° angle.
3. Place the right foot on the floor and repeat with the left leg.

Modified Jumping Jacks

1. Start in a standing position with the feet together and arms by the sides.
2. Tap right foot out to the side as the arms extend up to shoulder level.
3. Bring the right foot and arms back to starting position and repeat on the left side.

Pool Exercises (See Video for Exercise Examples)

These exercises can be completed in the shallow end or, for less impact, in the deep end of the pool holding a noodle or wearing a flotation belt.

Water Walking

1. Start in a standing position in shallow water with the feet flat on the floor, knees soft, abdominals engaged, and shoulders relaxed.
2. Walk across the pool floor, as if walking on land, placing the heel on the ground first and moving through to the ball of the foot.
3. Naturally move arms, placing the left arm forward when the right foot is stepping and right arm forward when the left leg is in front.

Knee Lifts

1. This exercise is similar to water walking except an added knee lift is incorporated before each footstep onto the floor.
2. Arms can move naturally or press against the water with each step.

Jumping Jacks

1. Start out standing in the pool with the feet together and arms by the side.
2. Slowly jump both feet out to the sides, rolling through the foot on the landing with the knees soft. Both arms extend out to the side but stay under the water.
3. Jump both feet back together and bring the arms back to the body.
4. Additional resistance can be added by starting with the arms in front of the body, parallel to the floor with palms together, and then extending the arms out to the side as both feet jump out.

Scissors

1. Start with feet hip-width apart with the right leg about 2–3 feet in front of the other. Knees are soft with the entire front foot on the floor and ball of the back foot on the floor. The left arm (opposite arm to the front leg) is in front and right arm slightly behind the torso.
2. Slowly jump and switch the arms and legs, landing softly with the left leg and right arm in front.

Balance Training

Many conditions associated with aging, including arthritis, muscle weakness, gait deficit, osteoporosis, and vision impairment, can lead to a loss of balance and stability [1]. This can in turn contribute to an increased risk for falls, fractures, injuries, and loss of physical function. Therefore, simple balance exercises should be incorporated into the exercise program to further develop core stability, muscle strength, and balancing skills. An improvement in these skills will not only reduce the risk for falls and injuries, but may also increase the older adult's confidence in the ability to perform activities of daily living and engage in an endurance exercise program.

Table 4.5 Ways to incorporate balance and coordination practice into everyday life

• Practice standing on one leg while performing daily tasks such as cleaning the dishes, combing hair, brushing teeth, or standing in line at the store
• When moving across a room, walk in a narrower stance (heel-to-toe), walk sideways, or walk with alternating knee lifts
• Try to stand up out of a chair without using hands
• Hold small objects out away from the body (while keeping elbows slightly bent) when walking

With some medical conditions, balance training may need to be completed before engaging in an endurance program, to ensure safety.

Balance exercises consist of positions or movements that challenge the individual to maintain posture and stability over a base of support. The ACSM recommends performing exercises that narrow the base of support, disrupt the center of gravity, stress postural muscles, or reduce sensory input [4]. Balance exercises completed 2–3 days/week can reduce the risk for falls and can be incorporated into an older adult's normal strength training program. Encourage the older adult to hold each balance position for 10–15 s, or for a length of time that is both challenging and safe to perform. Exercises can be completed near a wall, countertop, or a sturdy table or chair for assistance, especially for those who are just starting out or are at risk for falling. For more advanced progressions, balance exercises can be completed with the eyes closed or using a variety of equipment including balance pads, balance discs, small core balls, BOSU® balls, and stability balls.

Simple balance exercises can be incorporated into an older adult's daily activities with exercises that include standing on one foot while doing dishes or brushing teeth (Table 4.5). Balance exercises should be performed in sturdy shoes or bare feet. Having a sturdy object, such as a counter or table, to stand next to is important in case there is a loss of balance. Exercises based on the older adult's needs and abilities should be selected. Safety is a critical factor, and it is important for older adults to clear their environments of obstacles when performing balance training. If the older adult has poor balance or is nervous about trying the exercises, then he or she should perform the exercises with someone who could provide assistance. A cell phone or portable phone should also be within reach in case the older adult falls and needs help.

Balance Exercises

Balance Exercises
Single leg balance (see Fig. 4.31)

Single Leg Balance

1. Start in a standing position with the wall or a chair in front or to the side of body.
2. Gently place the hands against the wall or hold onto the edge of the chair.
3. Slowly lift the right foot off of the floor and place it to the front, side, or behind the body and hold for approximately 10-15 seconds.
4. Slowly place the foot back on the floor and lift the opposite leg.

   Progression

   - Release the hands from the chair or wall.
   - Slowly move the arms up over the head and then back down while balancing.
   - Close the eyes while performing this exercise.

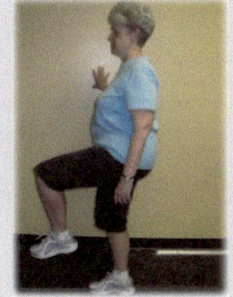

Fig. 4.31   Balance exercises. Single leg balance

Tandem standing (see Fig. 4.32)

Tandem Standing

1. Start in a standing position with the wall or chair for support if needed.
2. Place the right foot directly in front of the other with the right heel touching the left toes and hold this position for 10-15 seconds.
3. Repeat on the other side.

   Progression

   - Release the hands from the arm or chair and cross them over the chest.
   - Slowly move the arms above the head and then down or press a light medicine ball or weight above the head while holding this position.
   - Close the eyes.

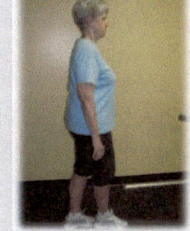

Fig. 4.32   Balance exercises. Tandem standing

Knee raises (see Fig. 4.33)

Knee Raises

1. Start out standing near a wall or chair for support if needed.
2. Slowly lift the right foot off the floor and raise the knee up until the hip is at a 90° angle.
3. Hold for 1-2 seconds and then slowly lower the foot down towards the floor until the foot is about an inch from touching the ground.
4. Without letting the right foot touch the floor, lift the right knee again and hold for 1-2 seconds again.
5. Repeat this 10 times on the right, trying to keep the right foot off of the floor throughout the exercise. Then repeat 10 times on the other side.

   Progression

   - This same exercise can be performed by raising the leg out to the side or extending the leg behind, not touching the floor between repetitions.

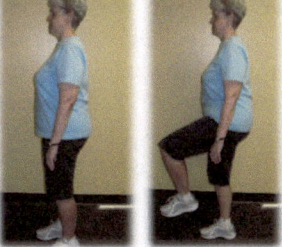

Fig. 4.33   Balance exercises. Knee raises

Stability ball sit (see Fig. 4.34)

Stability Ball Sit

1. Sit on top of a stability ball with the body centered on the ball and feet flat on the floor, hip-width apart.
2. Use the hands for support if needed by placing one hand on a chair or the wall.
3. Hold this seated position for 15-30 seconds or as long as possible.

   Progression
   - Add a leg lift by slowly lifting one foot off of the floor. Hold for 1-2 seconds and return to starting position.

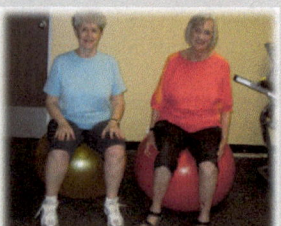

Fig. 4.34 Balance exercises. Stability ball sit

Moving Balance Exercises

- Alternate knee lifts while walking across the floor.
- Perform a tandem walk across the floor by placing each foot directly in front of the other in a toe-heel position.
- Place small blocks or cones on the floor, with approximately a foot and a half between each one. Slowly move forward across the floor, stepping over each block.
- With the blocks set up the same way as above, move sideways across the floor stepping over each block.

Additional Resources

In addition to the sample exercises mentioned throughout this chapter, structured exercise programs and classes designed specifically for older adults, such as tai chi, gentle or chair yoga, water aerobics, line dancing, Zumba Gold®, and the SilverSneakers Fitness® program are excellent ways to motivate and encourage older adults to exercise through a fun, supportive, and social environment. These classes are usually led by certified instructors who provide form and safety cues to ensure that class participants are performing the exercises correctly. Encourage older adults to visit the local YMCA, Senior Center, or other fitness facilities that offer specific programs for older adults.

Conclusion

Exercise plays a critical role in the maintenance and improvement in health, functional ability, and quality of life of the older adult. Medical professionals' opinions are valued by patients, and therefore can play a critical role in supporting and encouraging the older adult to become physically active. Be sure to ask the older adult detailed questions to determine his or her current level of fitness, readiness to participate in physical activity, and the activities he or she may enjoy. Any amount of time spent in physical activity is beneficial, whether it is exercising at home, walking outside, working out at a fitness center, participating in a sport, or joining a class. Therefore, encourage older adults to begin exercise programs that best fit their likes, needs, and goals.

References

1. American Geriatrics Society, British Geriatrics Society, and American Academy of Orthopaedic Surgeons Panel on Falls Prevention. Guideline for the prevention of falls in older persons. J Am Geriatr Soc. 2001;49(5):664–72.
2. Center for Disease Control and Prevention. How much physical activity do older adults need? 2001. Available from: http://www.cdc.gov/physicalactivity/everyone/guidelines/olderadults.html.
3. Izquierdo M, et al. International exercise recommendations in older adults (ICFSR): expert consensus guidelines. J Nutr Health Aging. 2021;25(7):824–53.
4. Liguori G, Feito Y, Fountaine C, Roy BA, editors. ACSM's guidelines for exercise testing and prescription. 11th ed. Philadelphia: Wolters Kluwer; 2022.
5. Nelson ME, Rejeski WJ, Blair SN, Duncan PW, Judge JO, King AC, Macera CA, Castaneda-Sceppa C. Physical activity and public health in older adults: recommendation from the American College of Sports Medicine and the American Heart Association. Med Sci Sports Exerc. 2007;39(8):1435–45.
6. Rikli R, Jones J. Senior fitness test manual. 2nd ed. Champaign: Human Kinetics; 2013.
7. Watt JR, Jackson K, Franz JR, Dicharry J, Evans J, Kerrigan DC. Effect of a supervised hip flexor stretching program on gait in frail elderly patients. Phys Med Rehabil. 2011;3(4):330–5.
8. Seguin R, Nelson ME. The benefits of strength training for older adults. Am J Prev Med. 2003;3(2):141–9.
9. Sallis R, Young DR, Tartof SY, Sallis JF, Sall J, Li Q, Smith GN, Cohen DA. Physical inactivity is associated with a higher risk for severe COVID-19 outcomes: a study in 48440 adult patients. Br J Sports Med. 2021;55:1099–105.

Chapter 5
Motivational Interviewing for Older Adults

Gail M. Sullivan, Alice K. Pomidor, and Kenneth Brummel-Smith

Key Points
- Motivational interviewing is a technique used to explore ambivalence about a behavior, such as physical activity
- Motivational interviewing uses open-ended questions, affirmations, reflections, and summarizations to help an older person self-analyze their behavior
- Motivational interviewing leads to modest improvements in physical activity in people with chronic health conditions
- There may be additional benefits to incorporating motivational interviewing into clinical practice
- The effects of motivational interviewing may be greater if the core components of motivational interviewing, such as open-ended questions, affirming what the patient says, providing reflections to link ideas, and summarizing, are used

Supplementary Information The online version contains supplementary material available at https://doi.org/10.1007/978-3-031-52928-3_5.

G. M. Sullivan (✉)
UConn Center on Aging, University of Connecticut School of Medicine,
Farmington, CT, USA
e-mail: gsullivan@uchc.edu

A. K. Pomidor
Florida State University (retired), Tallahassee, FL, USA
e-mail: apomidor@fsu.edu

K. Brummel-Smith
College of Medicine, Florida State University, Tallahassee, FL, USA
e-mail: ken.brummel-smith@med.fsu.edu

Case: Part 1
Mr. Jones is 75 years old and has hypertension, osteoarthritis of back and hips, obesity, and is now diagnosed as pre-diabetic. He has been told by several clinicians, over many years, that he needs to increase his physical activity and start an exercise program. He responds that he's never exercised and it's too late to start at his age. His primary clinician has retired and today he is going to see a new clinician, who plans to ask him questions about his motivations for not being active vs. being active.

Introduction

The majority of older persons do not engage in any regular physical activity program, although most are well aware of exercise benefits. Clinicians may feel frustrated when talking to patients about increasing their physical activity or starting an exercise program. Studies are inconclusive regarding whether making a recommendation to exercise, by itself, is effective in producing measurable patient benefits. Some of this uncertainty likely stems from clinicians infrequent use of evidence-based techniques for assisting patients to change long-standing habits and behaviors.

Motivational interviewing has emerged over several decades as an effective method to help individuals change behaviors. Motivational interviewing is a person-centered counseling style for helping older adults explore and resolve ambivalence about making behavior changes [1]. There is growing evidence documenting the effectiveness of motivational interviewing for increasing physical activity in older persons [2–6]. Studies are also examining the effectiveness of virtual motivational interviewing (VIMINT) which would enhance access to this strategy for older adults who live far from trained clinicians or have transportation problems [7]. In motivational interviewing, understanding an older adult's ambivalence is key to helping the older person make decisions to change an existing behavior.

Everyone has motivations for their behaviors. The older adult who does not exercise is either *motivated to do something other than exercise* or *motivated to not exercise*. However, virtually everyone—even most of those in the "precontemplative" stage of change—is also ambivalent about not exercising, as nearly everyone is aware that exercise is essential to good health. By focusing on and helping the individual to resolve this ambivalence, motivational interviewing increases the likelihood that the person will change a behavior.

Why would an older adult be motivated to maintain an unhealthy behavior? There are *always* disadvantages to change. Some healthy behaviors are seen as unpleasant, hard, or distasteful. Many people *enjoy* the status quo. They may feel, after a lifetime of hard work, it is their time to "rest" or that exercise is for younger persons. Others worry that they will not have the time to exercise or that they may be hurt if they start an exercise program. Some have limited resources to afford a gym or buy equipment, or may live in areas where outdoor walking is unsafe. The

Table 5.1 Ambivalent persons have big "buts"

I know I need to lose weight, *but* I hate exercising
I'd like to start walking, *but* I just don't have any time
I used to love swimming, *but* all those young women in their bathing suits make me feel self-conscious
I want to dance with my grandchildren, *but* I'm afraid I will fall

older adult who says "I'd like to start walking more, but I'm just too busy right now" is ambivalent. Listen carefully for the *but* in the statement that tells you the patient is ambivalent (Table 5.1). Exploring ambivalence is demonstrated in Video 5.1.

The Spirit of Motivational Interviewing

The "spirit" of motivational interviewing is different than the standard way most clinicians engage in discussions about behavior change. Most clinicians determine what are a patient's important problems and then give recommendations; clinicians see their role as experts providing advice and patient education. Motivational interviewing is collaborative rather than prescriptive. This technique recognizes that only in equal partnership with older adults can joint decision-making occur. It seeks to evoke from the person her own source of motivation, rather than telling the person something she must do. This strategy recognizes that we can never motivate someone else—motivation must come from within. Motivational interviewing honors autonomy. It recognizes that people generally resist when they are told to do something and feel respected when their viewpoints are elicited. A willingness to listen and learn is required when employing motivational interviewing. Some health care professionals, particularly physicians, are more comfortable giving orders to be followed rather than eliciting from the patient what matters most.

Motivation has traditionally been viewed as an internal personality trait. For example, people who do not exercise are lazy, nonadherent, or short-sighted. If motivation were actually an intrinsic personality trait, it would be difficult to change. The motivational interviewing approach views motivation as transactional: it depends on the relationship between two or more people, is temporary, and changes over time. Trying to make someone change when she has no interest or fears change is like getting into a wrestling match. Motivational interviewing is more like a dance. In this type of dancing, it is the older adult who does most of the leading.

Practitioners in medical encounters use three main types of communication styles: *directing, following, and guiding*. Directing the patient to do something is perhaps the most common form of communication used by health care professionals. The clinician takes charge, at least for the moment: "I'm going to start you on this medication for your blood pressure." The expected role of the patient is to learn from the information given by the clinician and adhere to the advice. In reality, this communication style is not very effective in many situations. The unequal power relationship may work well in a dire emergency, but it does little to facilitate long-standing behavior change. Providing knowledge alone rarely translates into changed behaviors. Often the prescriptive model initiates a wrestling match—the "yes, but" response from the older person.

The *following style* requires the clinician to suspend his own agenda and listen, very carefully, to the older adult's agenda. It is also the foundation of the patient-centered approach. In following the patient's lead, the clinician attempts to understand the patient's perspective. What are the older person's goals? How do those goals conflict with current behavior? What are the worries and concerns about change? Simple techniques such as nodding the head and saying "Uh-huh" and "Go on" allow the older adult to provide glimpses into the ambivalence he feels.

One can unwittingly set up roadblocks to listening. One has to avoid disagreeing, challenging, arguing, or shaming the person for what she has said. This will most certainly curtail the individual's comfort with discussing the difficulties of making a change. Similarly, too quickly agreeing with the person, expressing approval, or reassuring her may inhibit full disclosure. Silence while waiting a few seconds for the person to continue is usually the simplest method to use.

Guiding is perhaps the least utilized skill in traditional medical professional-patient interactions. A guide does not choose the outcome but can help with the journey. A key component of guiding is exploring options. For instance, in a person newly diagnosed with heart failure, an important step is to clarify the person's goals of care. Here the listening skill predominates. The older adult may reply that avoiding hospitalization and not taking too many medications are his goals. The proper response using motivational interviewing would be to ask, "Are you interested in learning about the ways to prevent hospitalizations and lessen the need for medications?" The door is now open to discuss physical activity, stress reduction, diet modifications, and other options.

The Process of Change

Change in behavior starts with ambivalence. If someone is completely committed to a certain course of behavior, there is nothing that the clinician can do. Often such committed persons are labeled as "resistant," "noncompliant," or "unmotivated." If an older adult is resisting the clinician's recommendations, it is a good sign that the current approach is not working and a change in course is needed. Doing *more* of what does not work will not work. In most cases, however, the person is not totally committed to the present course. In this situation the first step is a deeper exploration of the person's ambivalence. There are four useful techniques for engaging in discussions of motivation: using open-ended questions, affirming what the patient says, providing reflections to link ideas, and summarizing (OARS) (Table 5.2).

One can start by asking the older adult to describe the values or benefits she receives from her present behavior. For instance, if you were discussing sedentary behavior, you might ask, "What do you like about sitting at home each day?"

Table 5.2 OARS techniques

O	Open-ended questions
A	Affirmations
R	Reflections
S	Summarizing

Table 5.3 Change talk

"I don't know, I might be able to do it"
"I wish I could"
"I'll try to do it"
"I'll help if I can"
"I'll think about it"

Table 5.4 Using DARN to ask questions

Desire	What do you want, like, wish, or hope for?
Ability	What is possible? What can or could you do? What are you able to do first?
Reasons	Why would you make this change? What would be bad about it?
Need	How important is this change? Why do you need to do it?

(Open-ended question) This may seem counter-intuitive because we don't want to appear to be sanctioning "unhealthy behaviors." However, the question does not connote approval of the behavior, but rather shows respect for the person as a decision-maker. It is important not to cut off the person's listing of positive outcomes of his present behavior. Asking "What else?" or "I'm interested in hearing other important reasons you've had that prevented you going walking outside" shows the person that you are genuinely interested in what is really important to her. If the person says that she is so busy doing volunteer work that she cannot afford the time to exercise, one can use an affirmation to show that you respect her choice, "So, you really are very busy and successful in your volunteer work."

Open, nonjudgmental listening opens the door for the patient to engage in *change talk* (see Table 5.3). Motivational interviewing looks for themes in change talk. These themes can be remembered using the acronym, DARN—desire, ability, reasons, and need. Desire refers to a person's wish to change. Often the patient uses phrases like "I want...," I would like to...," or "I want to..." when engaging in change talk. Ability is more active and connotes that the patient can or should be able to do something. Reasons stated usually point to specific outcomes: to be able to play with grandchildren, to lose weight, etc. Change talk about needs often refers to how important the change is to the person. DARN can also be used to frame questions for greater clarification (see Table 5.4). Examples of these are found in Video 5.2.

The purpose of change talk is to develop *discrepancy* in the person's mind. People consider change when they become uncomfortable with the status quo. If the older adult views what is happening now in a relatively negative light compared to how he wants things to be, he will begin to examine conflicting motivations. The goal of this strategy is to enable the person to become aware of his deeper goals and values. A person may appreciate time gained to work on email by forgoing a 30-minute walk, but he may also more deeply value the benefit of weight loss. Ultimately it is the older adult, not the clinician, who should voice the arguments for change.

It is possible to elicit change talk, particularly in older adults who are contemplating a change in behavior. If you are the one bringing up exercise, it is always wise to ask permission, "Can I ask you some questions about exercise?" If the response is "no," then it is best to forgo further discussion. You may add, "If you change your mind, I'd be interested to hear your thoughts about it." This shows respect for the person and keeps the agenda focused on issues he wants to address. If the person responds positively and you know that the person does not engage in any regular physical activity, then begin with an open-ended question, "If you were to begin a regular activity program, what would you hope to see happen?" The use of a reflection can clarify the difficult choice the patient is making when faced with changing a behavior, "So, you've given a lot of thought to getting more physical activity, but you're also concerned how it might affect your health." A commonly used technique in motivational interviewing is the use of *rulers* to gage the importance of the change or the degree of confidence. For instance, after hearing change talk you can ask, "So, on a scale of 0, not important at all, to 10, very important, where would you put yourself regarding starting a walking program" (Fig. 5.1)? Someone scoring himself toward not being important is likely to be poorly motivated to change. Similarly, people with very low confidence that they will be able to start an exercise program may need much more interviewing about their competing motivations. Confidence can also be judged by using a "confidence scale" in the interview (Fig. 5.2). Regardless of where they score themselves, it is key to understand why they chose that number. A secondary question to ask is, "Why did you not give yourself a 3 instead of a 5 for importance?" This will help the individual

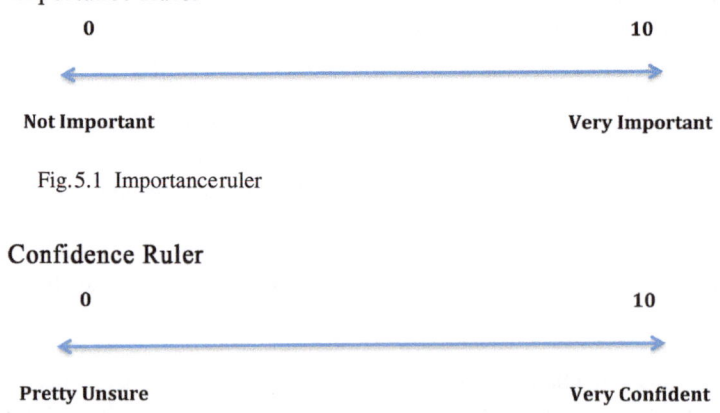

Importance Ruler

0   10

Not Important   Very Important

Fig.5.1 Importance ruler

Confidence Ruler

0   10

Pretty Unsure   Very Confident

Fig. 5.2 Confidence ruler

identify personal reasons for change. Similarly, asking the person who says his confidence level is a 6 why he didn't choose an 8 will enable her to explore perceived barriers to change. This is illustrated in Video 5.3.

Periodically *summarizing* what the person has said is another important technique used in motivational interviewing. Summarizations serve multiple purposes: showing that you have been listening, helping the patient to continue talking and possibly use change talk, and opening the door for gentle probing and clarification. By summarizing what has been said, the older adult also has the opportunity to correct any misunderstandings. That enables the individual to have a more equal status in the discussion. One can provide a simple summarization by repeating what was said. This is particularly important when change talk has occurred. For instance, when an older adult states she wants to start exercising because her mother had diabetes, never exercised, and had an amputation, you might say, "So, you don't want to end up like your mother who lost a leg to diabetes." Summarizing allows you to highlight or emphasize statements and to change direction.

Summarizations can also be used to draw different aspects of discussion together. For example, a patient may know that exercise would be good for him, but he is concerned that he may develop pain with a program such as walking. You might say, "So you feel that getting regular exercise would be helpful in helping control your high blood pressure, but you're afraid that starting to exercise could aggravate your arthritis." Summarizations are particularly helpful when a discussion has revealed various options, but the path ahead has not been decided. For example, "We've talked about your interest in starting a walking program and that it's pretty important to you and that your confidence is not high that you'll be able to stick with it. Where do we go from here?" This allows the older adult to be the one to initiate a plan, rather than the plan coming from the clinician. An example conversation is shown in Video 5.4.Informing the older adult is part of motivational interviewing as well, although it is much less directive than traditional medical interviewing. Perhaps the most significant difference is the importance of asking permission before providing information. This allows the clinician to play the role of the guide, rather than the drill sergeant. Asking permission honors the individual's autonomy and promotes more active involvement. The clinician and the older adult can then enter into a collaborative process, which lowers resistance to change. How to "roll with resistance" is demonstrated in Video 5.5.

There are many ways of asking permission. One example is, "Would you like to know what you could do for your joint pain?" After providing evidence-based options, you can follow the list with, "Would you like to hear more about any of these?" If a physical activity program is the choice, a follow-up question might be, "Would you like to hear about the benefits and risks of starting an exercise program?" Beware of overwhelming the person with information. The goal is not to "cover the material" but rather to help the older adult discover her conflicting motivations and gain more clarity about the direction she wants to follow.

Putting It Together

The most important aspect of motivational interviewing is the clinician's commitment to active listening. Listening is what distinguishes this type of interviewing most from traditional approaches to behavior change. Active listening suspends all judgment. It seeks to resist the "righting reflex"—the common response of trying to fix the person. It recognizes that if the clinician advocates for change, the individual may increase his resistance to change. Instead, the clinician must listen, very carefully, for the reasons why the older adult might think he wants to change. How important is change? Why would he want to do it? What are his worries about it? It is only by nonjudgmental listening that the individual's dormant motivation will come forth.

Through listening, the clinician is sometimes rewarded with DARN talk—what the person desires, how able she feels to change, the reasons why change might be worth pursuing, or the need that is driving the motivation. If this buried treasure is heard, the clinician can explore these areas. Sometimes rulers—how confident, how important is it to move toward a change in behavior—can then be used. These questions help to deepen the individual's desire and awareness of the need to change. Through these techniques ambivalence can be elicited and clarified. Working with the patient at all stages is illustrated in Videos 5.6 and 5.7.

Finally, after the reasons for change have been explored, the clinician may have the opportunity to inform the patient, with the patient's permission. Informing in motivational interviewing adheres to the concept that no one knows best, for we all know differently. No one can motivate another person. The real goal in motivational interviewing is to help older adults discover their own motivations and then support them in learning more about them.

Case: Part 2

Mr. Jone's new clinician asks him what he likes about staying at home, sitting most of the day. He responds that until retirement at 67, he worked extremely long, unpredictable hours in a factory: now he loves being completely in charge of his day. He knows exercise could help him, especially now that he's been told he may develop diabetes: he does not want to have diabetes! When asked what keeps him from being more active, he says, "I think I'd like going to the Y where a lot of my friends go, *but* I'm afraid I'll injure myself, hurt my joints." The clinician recognizes *ambivalence talk* and asks Mr. Jones if they can talk about this more. He is agreeable. From their discussion Mr. Jone's clinician perceives that the patient also lacks confidence; she summaries, "I hear that you care a lot about controlling your schedule and preventing diabetes, but you're not confident that you can avoid injuries if you are more active." They discuss the relative importance *to him* of being in control of his schedule, fear of pain, and avoiding diabetes, by using a gauge of 0 to 10. It turns out that these goals are all important, but improving pain and avoiding diabetes are the most important.

After engaging in *change talk* questions, the clinician asks, "Where do we go from here?" Mr. Jones responds that he wants to ask his friends about when the Y is open and Y programs. He asks, "Can we talk about this again, in a couple of weeks?"

References

1. Rollnick S, Miller WR. What is motivational interviewing? Behav Cogn Psychother. 1995;23:325–34.
2. O'Halloran PD, Blackstock F, Shields N, Holland A, Iles R, Kinglsey M, et al. Motivational interviewing to increase physical activity in people with chronic health conditions: a systematic review and meta-analysis. Clin Rehabil. 2014;28(12):1159–71.
3. Rubak S, Sandbaek A, Lauritzen T, Christensen B. Motivational interviewing: a systematic review and meta-analysis. Br J Gen Pract. 2005;55(513):305–12.
4. Knight KM, McGowan L, Dickens C, Bundy C. A systematic review of motivational interviewing in physical health care settings. Br J Health Psychol. 2006;11:319–32.
5. Chater AM, Schulz J, Jones A, Burke A, Carr S, Kukucska D, Troop N, Trivedi D, Howlett N. Outcome evaluation of active hearts: a community-based physical activity programme for inactive adults at risk of cardiovascular disease and/or low mental wellbeing. Front Public Health. 2022 Sep;9(10):903109.
6. Marina Arkkukangas M, Söderlund A, Eriksson S, Johansson A. One-year adherence to the Otago Exercise Program with or without motivational interviewing in community-dwelling older adults. J Aging Phys Act. 2018;26(3):390–5.
7. Motivational interviewing for physical activity among older adults. US National Library of Medicine. Clinical Trials.gov. https://clinicaltrials.gov/ct2/show/NCT05179148. Accessed 21 March 2023.

Resources

Motivational Interviewing Network of Trainers: www.motivationalinterviewing.org—a website with resource, references, videos, and links to training opportunities. Experienced motivational interviewers can be seen discussing the spirit of motivational interviewing and the way it work in videos. Accessed 21 March 2023.
Rollnick S, Miller WR, Butler CC. Motivational interviewing in health care: helping patients change behavior. New York: Guilford Press; 2008. An excellent resource for understanding the basics of motivational interviewing in a health care setting written by the founders of motivational interviewing.

Chapter 6
Writing an Exercise Prescription for Older Adults

Ashley L. Artese and Lynn B. Panton

Key Points
- As credible sources of health information, clinicians are in an ideal position to talk to their older adults about physical activity
- Rather than a "one size fits all" approach, designing an exercise program for older adults requires using medical conditions, health history, and physical function to guide the exercise prescription
- Use standard tests for strength, balance, endurance, and flexibility to assess the older adult's initial physical function, to tailor the exercise prescription and follow progress
- Four steps will guide the exercise program: (1) set goals; (2) choose exercises; (3) determine frequency, intensity, time, and type; and (4) follow principles of exercise prescription
- Exercise program design is a fluid process and will adjust over time to meet the needs of the older adult

Supplementary Information The online version contains supplementary material available at https://doi.org/10.1007/978-3-031-52928-3_6.

A. L. Artese (✉)
Department of Exercise Science and Health Promotion, Charles E. Schmidt College of Science, Florida Atlantic University, Boca Raton, FL, USA
e-mail: aartese@fau.edu

L. B. Panton
Florida State University, Tallahassee, FL, USA
e-mail: lpanton@fsu.edu

Introduction

Physical activity plays a key role in the prevention and clinical management of many chronic diseases. In addition, regular engagement in physical activity can reduce fall risk, improve physical function, and maintain activities of daily living (ADL) in older adults. Despite these benefits, the majority of older adults do not meet the current physical activity guidelines [1]. Health care professionals are important sources of information about the benefits of physical activity for their patients. Clinicians can provide counseling that is tailored to the older adult's conditions with ongoing feedback. For example, the measurements of body weight and blood pressure are measured at most clinician visits and respond favorably to physical activity. Increase in body weight or blood pressure can be detected at yearly well-check visits and lead to lifestyle discussions, including an exercise prescription. Furthermore, older adults report that a primary reason for starting or continuing participation in an exercise program is because their physician has told them to do so [2].

This chapter will provide resources and tools for clinicians to use in assessing an older adult's fitness level and encouraging physical activity. In addition, this chapter will discuss guidelines for writing an exercise prescription for the four exercise program components—endurance, strength, flexibility, and balance—to promote improvement in functional capacity and overall health in older adults.

Assessing Functional Fitness for Exercise Prescriptions

Depending on factors, such as age, chronic conditions, and current exercise habits, fitness level and functional ability will vary among older adults. Therefore, gathering information about medical conditions, health history, and physical function is essential when devising an appropriate exercise prescription tailored to the older adult. While a clinician should already have information regarding the patient's medical and health history, additional assessments to measure endurance, strength, flexibility, and balance may be needed. There are several functional tests specific to older adults that can be easily performed, with minimal time and equipment, by a nurse, medical assistant, or other personnel. These tests include the Short Physical Performance Battery (SPPB) [3], Senior Fitness Test [4, 5], six-minute walk test (6MWT) [6], 3 or 4 or 10 m walk [3, 7], and single leg stance test (Table 6.1). Normative values for these tests are available for older adults along with chronic disease-specific standardized scores. Benefits of administering one or more of these assessments prior to prescribing an exercise program include:

- Identifying physical limitations and safety concerns that should be considered when designing the exercise program

Table 6.1 Functional fitness assessments for older adults

Test	Description	Administration time	Scoring
Short physical performance battery (SPPB)	Assesses lower body function using tests for balance, gait speed, and chair stands Equipment – Stopwatch – Chair without arms (seat height: 17″)	10 min	Score range: 0–12 – Higher scores indicate better function – Score ‹10 indicates functional limitations
Senior fitness test[a]	Assesses aerobic capacity, upper and lower body function, balance, and flexibility using these tests: 30-s chair stand, 30-s arm curl, 6 m walk test, 2-min step test, chair sit and reach, back scratch, and 8-foot up and go Equipment – Stopwatch – Chair without arms (seat height: 17″) – Hand weights (5-lb and 8-lb) – Cone	30 min – Each test requires 2–10 min	Normative values available for each test – Scores ≤25 percentile for each age group are considered below average
Six-minute walk test (6MWT)	Assesses functional aerobic capacity by measuring the distance the older adults can walk in 6 min Equipment – Stopwatch – Cones to mark track – Measuring wheel	8–10 minutes	Normative values and equations for VO_{2max} (maximal oxygen consumption) prediction available for recorded distance
Single leg stance	Assesses balance by measuring time held for a single leg balance Equipment – Stopwatch	1–2 min	Normative values available
3, 4, or 10 m walk test (walking speed)	Assesses gait velocity, functional ability, and balance Equipment: – Stopwatch – Measured distance	1–2 min	Normative values available

[a] For videos of the senior fitness test battery, see Chap. 4

- Identifying specific movements and/or functional limitations to use for focusing the exercise prescription to improve functional performance in high priority domains or to prevent further declines in specific areas
- Providing feedback to older adults about their strengths and areas for improvement

- Developing an individualized exercise prescription that is specific to the older adult's needs, functional ability, and goals
- Obtaining a baseline measurement to evaluate improvement in fitness, strength, and physical function over time
- Evaluating the effectiveness of the prescribed exercise program

Choosing a Functional Fitness Assessment

To determine which functional fitness assessments to use, consider:

Time and Feasibility

The administration of functional fitness assessments to older adults can range from 1 to 30 min depending on the specific tests chosen and the number of tests administered. Choose tests that are both feasible to conduct in the clinical setting and fit within the time allotted for the appointment.

Appropriateness of the Test

Consider the older adult's overall health and function when deciding which tests to administer. For example, the SPPB may be appropriate for older adults with poor health and low functional ability, but it may not be challenging enough for higher functioning older adults who may achieve the maximum score on the test. Due to this ceiling effect, the test would be limited in detecting improvement over time. Therefore, the Senior Fitness Test Battery, 6MWT, and single leg stand may be more appropriate for higher functioning older adults.

Alignment of Test with Appropriate Domain

Choose the functional test that aligns with the domain of interest. For example, if the clinician wants to obtain information regarding the older adult's endurance, the 2-min step test or the 6MWT would be most appropriate since they are indicators of cardiorespiratory fitness. Table 6.2 illustrates which functional tests align with each exercise domain.

Table 6.2 Exercise domains and aligned assessments

Exercise domain	Assessment
Endurance	• 6MWT (SFT) • 2-minute step test (SFT)
Strength	• Chair stand (SPPB) • 30-second chair stand (SFT) • 30-second arm curl (SFT)
Balance and mobility	• Balance tests—single leg, semi-tandem, and tandem stand (SPPB) • Gait speed (SPPB) • 8-foot up and go (SFT) • Single leg stance • 3, 4, or 10 meter walk
Flexibility	• Chair sit and reach (SFT) • Back scratch (SFT)

6MWT six-minute walk test, *SFT* senior fitness test, *SPPB* short physical performance battery

Designing the Exercise Prescription

After gathering medical, health, and functional information about the older adult, the next step is to determine the components to be included in the exercise program. A comprehensive, well-rounded exercise program should consist of four components: *endurance, strength, flexibility, and balance*. For older adults who demonstrate minimal functional limitations and are already physically active, an exercise program consisting of two or more of these components can be initially prescribed, with the goal of integrating all four components into the program over time. For older adults with low or impaired physical function, first focus on balance and/or strength components by using supported exercises, such as holding onto a chair or walker, along with flexibility training for range of motion. Endurance exercises such as walking or other unsupported weight-bearing exercises can be added later. Once the initial components to be included in the exercise prescription are determined, the exercise program for the older adult can be designed using these four steps.

Step 1: Set Goals

Prior to designing the exercise program, take several minutes to discuss the importance of exercise and the health benefits the older adult can obtain. Then, determine prior or current experiences with exercise, and identify one to two initial goals related to the older adult's health history, functional assessment results, and personal goals. In addition, discuss potential barriers or challenges to exercise adherence the older adult may experience. Use effective strategies to set goals, overcome barriers, and prepare the older adult for engagement in the exercise program.

Set SMART Goals Encourage the older adult to set goals that are **S**pecific, **M**easurable, **A**ttainable, **R**elevant to his or her values, and **T**ime-specific. Goals should be detailed with outcomes that can be measured and assessed over time to track improvement. An attainable and realistic time frame to achieve each goal should be established. Goals can be related to health outcomes (e.g., blood pressure or blood glucose values), performance on functional assessments (e.g. increasing number of chair stands or touching toes), or behavior (e.g., completing three exercise sessions per week for the next month) (See Box 6.1).

Develop an Action Plan Once SMART goals have been determined, establish an action plan with steps for achieving those goals. These steps can consist of weekly behavioral targets (e.g., walk for 20 min three times per week during weeks 1 and 2 of the exercise program) or bi-weekly or monthly benchmarks (e.g., complete 150 min of walking per week for 4 weeks). Creating an action plan with weekly behavioral targets or short-term benchmarks helps break goals into smaller manageable steps, increase motivation, and build patient self-efficacy for exercise.

Develop Specific Strategies to Overcome Barriers After identifying potential barriers or challenges that may negatively influence adherence to the exercise program, establish feasible ways to overcome these challenges. Strategies can include creating shorter workouts for days when time is limited, walking inside at the mall when it is raining, determining exercise modifications that accommodate symptoms related to chronic diseases, and identifying a potential exercise buddy to provide social support (see Chap. 5 for additional motivation interviewing strategies).

Box 6.1 Designing a SMART Goal

Example: A 30-second chair test and 30-second arm curl test were administered to a 75-year-old male older adult. He completed eight chair stands (interpretation: below average) and 18 arm curls (interpretation: average). After the clinician and patient discuss the results and the patient's values they decide that a suitable goal is to improve lower body physical function, which will help to prevent further lower body weakness and may prevent future falls. Normative values for the chair stand test for his age group is 11–17 chair stands. Based on this information, the following SMART goals are established:

SMART Goal #1 (Performance Goal): The goal is to improve the 30-s chair stand test score from 8 repetitions to 15 repetitions by the end of 12-weeks.

SMART Goal #2 (Behavioral Goal): The goal is to complete the prescribed strength training program (6 strength exercises completed for two sets of 10–15 repetitions) two times per week for the next 12 weeks.

Step 2: Choose the Exercises

Choosing exercises for the older adult's exercise program should not be a "one size fits all" approach. Instead, a variety of factors should be considered to ensure the exercises are safe and tailored to suit the specific needs and interests of the older adult. Start with determining which exercise components (endurance, strength, flexibility, and balance) will be included in the exercise program; once this has been established, exercise options specific to each component should then be considered. For example, if the program will include an endurance component, choose an exercise mode that is endurance-based (e.g., exercise that involve continuous movement of large muscle groups to elevate the heart rate, such as walking, cycling, or swimming). If the program will include a strength component, exercises that focus on building strength by challenging the muscles against an external resistance (e.g., leg press, chest press, biceps curls) should be considered. The flexibility component should consist of stretching exercises to improve range of motion. A balance component should include static exercises and dynamic movements that challenge the older adult to maintain posture and stability over a base of support. Chapter 4 provides specific exercise examples along with pictures and descriptions for each exercise component. Additional factors to consider when choosing exercises include appropriateness of the exercise and personal goals, safety, and feasibility.

Appropriateness of Exercise Determine exercises that are appropriate for the older adult's functional level and align with his or her goals. Use the information gathered from the health history, medical history, and/or functional assessments to guide the initial exercise prescription, as well as the patient's own goals. For example, if the older adult's performance on the 30-second chair stand test was below average and the patient wants to improve getting up to walk to the bathroom, a goal may be to improve lower body strength and function. In this case a focus on exercises that challenge the lower body such as chair stands, step-ups, and leg extensions match this goal. Older adults especially benefit from functional exercises that mimic everyday activities, such as climbing stairs, standing up from a chair, or bending down to pick up an object from the floor. Build confidence by selecting a few exercises that the older adult can perform well and focus on increasing functional capacity by prescribing exercises that challenge the older adult in areas where improvement is most needed.

Sometimes the patient's goal—such as to lose weight—may not match the most concerning functional assessment findings—poor balance with recurrent falls. When initiating a program, it is essential to respond to the patient's own goals; any exercise program a patient will do is better than no exercise at all. In the above case, pool-based endurance exercise may meet the patient's goals, without risking falls. In the future, program adjustments or additions can focus on patient-specific functional deficits.

In addition to prescribing exercises based on gathered information, consider how physical limitations, medications, and disease-related symptoms may affect the older adult's ability to perform certain exercises. For example, an older adult with obesity or osteoarthritis may experience joint pain while performing weight-bearing exercises, and therefore prescribing non-weight-bearing activities, like cycling or water exercise, may be better tolerated. Seated or supported exercises may be more appropriate for older adults who have poor balance or are taking medications, such as psychoactive and antihypertensive medications, associated with increased fall risk. Finally, contraindications associated with specific conditions or chronic diseases should be avoided. For example, kneeling exercises are not recommended following a knee replacement and sudden movements that involve bending, twisting, or compression of the spine should be avoided in individuals with osteoporosis.

Safety Safety is key when choosing the most appropriate exercises for the older adult's exercise program. The goal is to prescribe exercises that provide the most benefit, but can be performed safely with minimal risk. Older adults should be provided guidance on the safe use of equipment and proper technique for each exercise. Safety precautions relating to exercise selection should include: (1) minimizing fall risk by prescribing some seated exercises and encouraging older adults to perform standing or balancing exercises next to a wall or chair for support if needed; (2) reducing tripping hazards by limiting the amount of equipment needed to one or two items and confirming that the older adult has a space with adequate room and lighting to perform the exercise program; and (3) considering how the number and order of exercises may cause fatigue. It is recommended to work larger muscle groups and more complex movements first followed by single joint exercises for smaller muscle groups. Exercises involving larger muscle groups and complex movements are more challenging and require more energy, so prescribe them early in the workout. Technique and safety may be compromised if performed when an older adult is fatigued. Structure the exercise sequence with a combination of standing and seated exercises to manage leg fatigue and consider prescribing balance exercises earlier in the workout when the leg muscles are fresh to minimize fall risk.

Feasibility Choose exercises that are feasible to perform based on the available space and equipment. If the older adult plans to exercise at a fitness facility, exercises using cardio machines, weight machines, dumbbells, and other free weight equipment can be prescribed. If a home-based program is planned, inquire about availability of equipment. Resistance bands and dumbbells are inexpensive and portable for home-based programs. A set of stairs and household items including water bottles, milk jugs, soup cans, and towels can be used instead of purchasing equipment. Always prescribe exercises based on the older adult's preference for mode, equipment, and exercise location.

Step 3: Determine Frequency, Intensity, Time, and Type (FITT) for Each Component

The FITT principle outlines the important aspects of an exercise program design: frequency, intensity, time, and type. In order to tailor the exercise program to the specific needs of the older adult, each of these elements needs to be carefully considered and defined in the exercise prescription. *Frequency* is defined as the number of exercise sessions prescribed in a given time frame such as the number of sessions per week. *Intensity* refers to the amount of energy expended while performing an exercise. Intensity can be characterized in a variety of ways including heart rate, rating of perceived exertion (RPE), weight lifted, and difficulty of the exercise. *Time* indicates the duration of exercise or the components that determine the time required for the training session, such as number of exercises, repetitions, and sets. *Type* refers to the specific mode or movement of exercise being prescribed, such as walking, swimming, cycling, or stairclimbing. FITT guidelines for older adults have been established by the American College of Sports Medicine (ACSM) for each component of exercise.

FITT Prescription for Endurance Endurance or aerobic training involves the continuous movement of major muscle groups such as the legs and/or arms, to maintain an elevated heart rate for an extended period of time. Regular engagement in endurance exercise leads to increased cardiorespiratory fitness, improved ability to perform activities of daily living, and reduced fatigue during prolonged exercise or activity [8]. The US 2018 Physical Activity Guidelines for Americans [9] recommends that older adults accumulate 150–300 min of moderate-intensity aerobic activity per week, 75–150 min of vigorous-intensity aerobic activity, or a combination of the two. Moderate-intensity exercise is characterized as activity that causes an individual to breathe more than at rest or break a sweat, but able to talk and carry on a conversation. Vigorous-intensity activity is characterized by more rapid breathing and the ability to say a few words, but not carry on a continuous conversation without stopping for breath. The same endurance training mode can be altered to achieve moderate- or vigorous-intensity activity. For example, the intensity for walking can be increased from moderate to vigorous by increasing walking speed or grade. The ACSM provides detailed recommendations regarding endurance exercise, with these FITT guidelines [10]:

- Frequency: older adults should participate in endurance exercise 3–5 days/week. Consider intensity when prescribing frequency:

  - 5 days/week for moderate-intensity activity
  - 3 days/week for vigorous-intensity activity
  - 3-5 days/week for a combination of moderate- and vigorous-intensity activity

- Intensity: intensity should be prescribed based on relative fitness level or a 0–10 rating of perceived exertion (RPE) scale, where "0" represents no exertion and

"10" represents maximal exertion. Moderate- and vigorous-intensity activity should be prescribed based on:

– Moderate-intensity activity: RPE of 5–6
– Vigorous-intensity activity: RPE of 7–8

• Time: recommended time ranges from 20 to 60 min/day and can be accomplished during one continuous exercise bout or through several short exercise bouts throughout the day. When prescribing exercise time, prescribed intensity should be considered:

– Moderate-intensity activity: 30–60 min/day
– Vigorous-intensity activity: 20–30 min/day

• Type: older adults can choose any activity that raises the heart rate and involves continuous movement of large muscle group, such as walking, cycling, swimming, dancing, or an aerobic-based group exercise classes. Activity type should be chosen based on preference, safety, and tolerance for weight-bearing activities.

FITT Prescription for Strength Strength training, also known as weight or resistance training, involves the contraction of a muscle against a weight or type of resistance to build or maintain the strength and endurance of the muscle. Strength training can include exercises using body weight, weight machines, free weights, resistance bands, medicine balls, kettlebells, or other pieces of equipment that provide resistance. Strength exercises targeting these major muscle groups should be prescribed: quadriceps, hamstrings, gluteal muscles, calves, chest, upper back, shoulders, biceps, triceps, abdominals, and low back. The 2018 Physical Activity Guidelines for Americans recommends that older adults participate in strength training activities at least two days per week [9]. Specific FITT ACSM strength recommendations are [10]:

• Frequency: strength training should be performed on ≥2 days/week
• Intensity: intensity commonly refers to the amount of weight lifted, but it can also indicate the difficulty of the exercise. Weight is generally prescribed based on a percentage of one-repetition maximum (1RM), which is the maximum weight that can be lifted one time through a full range of motion. Recommended percentages range from 40–50% of 1RM when beginning a strength training program, which can progress to 60–80% of 1RM. Since 1RM tests are not commonly assessed in a clinical setting and require both time and equipment, intensity can be prescribed based on RPE or number of repetitions:

– RPE-based intensity: begin by prescribing a weight or difficulty level that is equivalent to an RPE of 5–6. Older adults can work up to an intensity that is equivalent to an RPE of 7–8 as tolerated.
– Prescribed repetitions: prescribe a weight that the older adult can lift safely with moderate exertion for a specific number of repetitions (10–15 repetitions).

- Time: time designated for the strength training prescription is determined by three factors:
  - Number of exercises: exercises focusing on the major muscle groups of the upper (approximately 6 to 8 exercises) and lower body (approximately 4 to 6 exercises)
  - Repetitions: 10–15 repetitions
  - Sets: 1–3 sets with a rest period of 1–2 min between sets
- Type: Any exercises that require older adults to work against a resistance can be prescribed, such as body weight, resistance band, weight machine, free weight, or water-based exercises.

FITT Prescription for Flexibility Flexibility training involves moving a joint through its range of motion with dynamic (with movement) and static (holding the position) movements to stretch muscles. Flexibility training prevents injury and joint pain, increases range of motion, and improves posture. Dynamic stretches are done during the warm-up to prepare the muscles for exercise and gradually increase range of motion. Dynamic stretches include stationary or walking knee lifts, half squats, and non-weighted arm movements such as shoulder raises. Dynamic stretches should be completed for 5–10 repetitions each. Static stretches, movements that are held for a certain length of time, are prescribed at the end of the workout to increase flexibility. The FITT ACSM stretching recommendations for older adults are [10]:

- Frequency: training should be performed 2 or more days per week, with greater benefits achieved with daily stretching
- Intensity: stretches should be held at the point where there is a slight discomfort in the muscle, without pain
- Time: stretches for all major muscle groups should be prescribed. Each stretch should be performed for 3–4 sets and held for 30–60 s
- Type: in static stretching the stretched position is held without movement or bouncing

FITT Prescription for Balance Balance training, also known as neuromotor training, involves exercises that challenge the older adults' ability to stabilize the body and maintain posture. Unstable surfaces, narrowing bases of support, weight shifts, or the removal of upper body assistance are used. Exercises that target mobility can also be included. Balance training can be prescribed as an individual training component, or for older adults with higher physical function, balance exercises can be incorporated into other training components. For example, balance challenges are integral to usual aerobic dance movements. Balance exercises could be incorporated during the rest period between two strength training exercise sets. Another option is to narrow the base of support while performing a standing upper body exercise, such as biceps curls, via standing with feet together or in a semi-tandem stance (feet place together, one half-way up the side of the other) during the set. Dynamic strength training also inherently trains balance as it challenges the ability to maintain stability while shifting body position over a base of support. Although FITT guidelines have not been established for balance training, general recommendations include [10]:

- Exercises that gradually narrow the base of support, such as moving from a two-legged stand to a single leg stand
- Dynamic movements that challenge the center of gravity, such as 90° or 180° turns, or walking in a figure-8 pattern
- Weight shifts or balance exercises that challenge posture, such as holding a calf raise or standing on an unstable surface
- Reducing sensory input, such as reducing lighting or closing eyes during an exercise
- Tai chi classes

Exercise Prescription and FITT Considerations

Although the FITT guidelines are valuable evidence-based recommendations to inform exercise program design, they may not be a realistic starting point for individuals with functional limitations, sedentary habits, or no experience with exercise programs. For these persons, starting frequency, intensity, and time should be at or below the lower end of the recommended ranges. Encourage the older adult to begin slowly and do what he or she is able to safely tolerate, with gradual progression over time. "Start low and go slow" is a useful mantra when advising older adults. Functional assessment results can inform the starting prescription decisions. For example, the completion of eight repetitions on the 30-s chair stand test indicates an appropriate starting repetition number of 8. Prior to beginning the exercise program, a warm-up consisting of 5–10 min of slow aerobic activity and dynamic movements should be incorporated, to gradually increase heart rate, body temperature, and joint movement. A cool-down with activities to gradually decrease the heart rate should be performed at the end of each training session. Often this will consist of the flexibility training component of the program.

Step 4: Follow the Principles of Exercise Prescription

After establishing goals, choosing exercises, and writing the FITT prescription, the final step is to consider the principles of exercise prescription to ensure safety and promote gradual improvement over time. These principles include *individualization, specificity, overload, progression, and reversibility*. Individualization refers to the development of an exercise program based on the individual's characteristics including age, health and medical history, functional level, exercise experience, goals, and preferences. Tailoring the exercise prescription to the specific needs of the older adult ensures that the program is safe, appropriate, and feasible.

The principle of specificity defines training-related adaptations as being specific to the type of movement performed and muscles trained. Therefore, the exercises in the program must be specific to the exercise components, functional movements, and specific muscles that the program is targeting to improve. For example, if the goal is to increase the ability to climb a flight of stairs, exercises that mimic stair climbing and increase strength of the hip flexors, quadriceps, hamstrings, gluteal muscles, and calves should be prescribed.

Overload refers to the necessity of prescribing exercises that challenge the older adult to do more work, in order to improve. Overload can be applied by increasing frequency, weight, repetitions, sets, and time as well as prescribing a more challenging variation of the exercise.

The progression principle refers to the need to gradually progress over time as the muscles and body adapt to the training load. Progression for endurance training uses the 10% rule; one FITT component is progressed by 10% every 1–2 weeks. For example, the prescribed time of the endurance activity can be increased from 20 min to 22 min every 1–2 weeks, as 2 min is 10% of 20. For strength training, the frequency, weight, repetitions, or sets can be increased, or a more advanced variation of the exercise can be prescribed. Balance can be progressed by continuing to narrow the base of support or reduce sensory input. Flexibility can be progressed by increasing the frequency, time, or type of stretch.

The final principle, reversibility, refers to the loss of exercise gains that occurs when exercise is discontinued. If participation in the exercise program is stopped for a period of time, the most recent training frequency, intensity, and time may need to be reduced when the program is restarted, to accommodate the loss in functional fitness that often occurs.

Putting It All Together

Using these four steps can help clinicians design a safe, appropriate, and feasible exercise program that is tailored to the specific needs of the older adult. Table 6.3 provides an example of how to use the four steps to design an exercise program. (See Data 6.1 for a sample exercise handout that can be given to the older adult.) Keep in mind that designing an exercise program is a fluid process in which the exercises and FITT prescription will be modified based on tolerance, changes in health or functional status, or the older adult's perceptions of and adherence to the program. The most successful exercise program is one that an older adult will do, thus, devising a program that works for the individual person is best. Participating in some exercise is always more beneficial than doing none at all.

Table 6.3 Sample exercise program using the four steps to design an exercise prescription

Sample exercise program
Example: A 30-s chair stand, 30-s arm curl, 2-min step test, and chair sit and reach (Senior Fitness Test battery) were administered to a 75-year-old woman. She completed 9 chair stands (below average), 14 arm curls (average), 65 steps on the 2-minute step test (below average), and a +1 on the chair sit and reach test (average). After the clinician and older woman discuss the assessments, the clinician decides that the exercise program should start with three exercise components (strength, endurance, and flexibility) and they jointly decide on two strength, one endurance, and one flexibility goal

SMART Goal #1: to improve the 30-s chair stand test score from 9 repetitions to 14 repetitions by the end of 12 weeks

SMART Goal #2: to improve the 30-s arm curl test score from 14 repetitions to 18 repetitions by the end of 12 weeks

SMART Goal #3: to improve the 2-min step test score from 65 steps to 85 steps by the end of the 12 weeks

She prefers to exercise at home and has light dumbbells available

	Step 1: goals	Step 2: choosing exercises[a]	Step 3: FITT prescription
Strength training	Goal #1: increase chair stand from 9 to 14 repetitions	Chair stand	**– F:** 2 days/week **– I:** RPE of 5–6 **– T:** 10–15 repetitions, 1 set **– T:** Bodyweight exercises
		Step-ups on a step	
	Goal #2: increase arm curl from 14 to 18 repetitions	Chest press (dumbbells)	
		Upright row (dumbbells)	
		Front shoulder raise (dumbbells)	
		Biceps curl (dumbbells)	
		Triceps Extension (dumbbells)	
Endurance training	Goal #3: increase 2-min step test performance from 65 steps to 85 steps	Walking	**F:** 3 days/week **I:** RPE of 5–6 **T:** 20 min **T:** Outdoor walking

Step 4: principles of exercise prescription

- **Individualization:** The exercise prescription was designed with the older adult's goals, functional level, and equipment needs in mind
- **Specificity:** Prescribed exercises align with the goals
- **Overload and progression:** The program starts at moderate intensity with low frequency and time. FITT will be gradually progressed every 1–2 weeks to ensure progressive overload
  - The program starts with two exercise components (strength and endurance). Over time, flexibility and balance training can be added to create a more comprehensive program
- **Reversibility:** The older adult will be encouraged to complete the prescribed program weekly. Adjustments will be made if the program needs to be restarted following discontinuation

[a] See Chap. 4 for pictures and descriptions of all the exercises listed in the table, *F* Frequency, *I* Intensity, *T* Time, *T* Type

Resources

These resources have more information regarding functional fitness testing, exercise prescription, and programs specific to older adults.

Functional Fitness Assessment Tools

- **The National Institute of Health (NIH) Toolbox** (https://nihtoolbox.force.com/s/article/nih-toolbox-administrators-manual-and-elearning-course)

  The NIH Toolbox is a standard set of valid, reliable, and royalty-free tools for assessing cognitive, emotional, motor, and sensory functions in older adults. The NIH Toolbox measures have been normed and validated across the age ranges from 3 to 85 years of age. Physical function tests include a 4-meter walk gait speed test for locomotion, 2-min walk test for endurance, standing balance test, 9-hole pegboard test for dexterity, and handgrip test for strength.

- **Senior Fitness Test or Fullerton Functional Test** (https://www.topendsports.com/testing/senior-fitness-test.htm)

  The Senior Fitness test, developed by Drs. Roberta Rikli and Jessie Jones, is simple and assesses the functional fitness of adults 60 years and above. This battery of tests has performance scores and normative data from 7000 men and women ages 60–94 years. The test battery includes a 30-s chair stand test for lower body strength, 30-s arm curl test for upper body strength, chair sit and reach test for lower body flexibility, 8-foot up and go test for agility, and two endurance tests—the 6-min walk test or the 2-min step in place test.

  Rikli, R. E., & Jones, C. J. (2013). Senior fitness test manual. Human kinetics.

- **Short Physical Performance Battery**

  https://www.nia.nih.gov/research/labs/leps/short-physical-performance-battery-sppb

- **Short Physical Performance Battery Guide:** www.sppbguide.com

  The National Institute on Aging provides instructions, videos, and resources for administering the Short Physical Performance Battery.

- **Six-minute Walk Test Instructions**

- **American Thoracic Society Statement: Guidelines for the Six-Minute Walk Test:** ATS Committee on Proficiency Standards for Clinical Pulmonary Function Laboratories. (2002). ATS statement: guidelines for the six-minute walk test. Am J Respir Crit Care Med, 166, 111-117. https://doi.org/10.1164/ajrccm.166.1.at1102

- **Single Leg Stance Protocol**

  Springer BA, Marin R, Cyhan T, Roberts H, Gill NW. Normative values for the unipedal stance test with eyes open and closed. J Geriatr Phys Ther. 2007;30(1):8–15.

Facility Based, On-line, and Manuals of Exercise Programs for the Older Adult

- **Exercise is Medicine** (https://www.exerciseismedicine.org)

  Exercise is Medicine (EIM) is a global health initiative by the American College of Sports Medicine (ACSM) and the American Medical Association (AMA) in response to the overwhelming evidence of the therapeutic role of physical activity in the prevention and management of chronic diseases. EIM's vision is to make physical activity assessment and promotion a standard in clinical care. A primary objective of EIM is to for clinicians to include a physical activity question as a vital sign and recommend physical activity as a prescription, just like they would do for a medication.

  There are many resources for physicians and patients at the EIM website, such as the Health Care Providers' Action Guide (https://www.exerciseismedicine.org/wp-content/uploads/2021/02/EIM-Health-Care-Providers-Action-Guide-clickable-links.pdf), which contains the Physical Activity Vital Sign, Exercise is Medicine Rx form, Rx for Health Series patient handouts, Community Resources handout template, and Provided Coding and Billing Tips. The Rx for Health Series includes handouts in English and Spanish for exercise prescriptions for 30 different diseases and conditions, such as Alzheimer's dementia, heart failure, and hypertension. Directions for the exercise prescription and examples of activities are simple and limited to three pages.

- **SilverSneakers® by Tivity Health** (https://tools.silversneakers.com/)

  SilverSneakers® is a US community wellness program established to help older adults 65 years and older take control of their health. The program includes live online fitness classes, on-demand videos, and access to thousands of gyms across the country. There are a variety of physical and wellness activities for strength, endurance, and flexibility training.

- **Renew Active®** (https://www.uhc.com/member-resources/health-care-programs/wellness-and-rewards-programs/renew-active)

  UnitedHealthcare replaced SilverSneakers® with Renew Active®, which is similar to SilverSneakers®. This program offers a list of participating gyms and fitness centers which can be accessed on their website through Find a Fitness Location (https://www.uhcrenewactive.com/location). Renew Active® is a fitness program designed to keep body and mind fit. The program is available with select UnitedHealthCare Medicare Advantage plans and includes memberships at participating fitness facilities at no extra cost, as well as online exercises and activities for brain health.

- **American Heart Association** (https://www.heart.org/?s_src=22U5W1AEMG&s_subsrc=evg_sem&gclid=EAIaIQobChMI86Ok_OTf-QIVKcmUCR01uACWEAAYASAAEgINvPD_BwE&gclsrc=aw.ds)

  The American Heart Association is a national, non-profit organization dedicated to the reduction of death and disability from cardiovascular diseases and stroke. Their website has healthy eating guidelines and exercise programs (https://www.heart.org/en/healthy-living/fitness/fitness-basics) and books that can be downloaded.

- **National Institute of Health (NIH) and National Institute of Aging (NIA)** (https://www.nia.nih.gov/health/exercise-physical-activity)

  The National Institute of Aging (NIA) leads scientific efforts to understand the nature of aging and extend the healthy, active years of life for older adults. Their website has articles such as how to get started exercising, real-life benefits, staying motivated, finding the right fitness clothes, safety tips for exercising outdoors, exercising with chronic conditions, and exercise and physical activity tracking tools. These resources are printed in English and Spanish. Their book, *Get Fit for Life: Exercise & Physical Activity for Health and Aging,* can be downloaded or ordered free of charge from the website (https://order.nia.nih.gov/publication/get-fit-for-life-exercise-physical-activity-for-healthy-aging).

- **U.S. Department of Health and Human Services** (https://health.gov/our-work/nutrition-physical-activity/move-your-way-community-resources/campaign-materials/materials-older-adults)

  U.S. Department of Health and Human Services developed the Move Your Way® campaign to help older adults learn about exercise benefits and find activities that work for them. Resources on their website include videos, interactive tools, and downloadable PDFs.

- **American Association of Retired Persons (AARP)** (https://www.aarp.org/)

  AARP is the nation's largest nonprofit, nonpartisan organization dedicated to empowering older adults. AARP focuses on health security, financial stability, and personal fulfillment. Members of AARP have access to exercise videos (https://www.aarp.org/search/?q=Exercise&c=everywhere).

References

1. National Center for Health Statistics. Table 25: Participation in leisure-time aerobic and muscle-strengthening activities that meet the federal 2008 Physical Activity Guidelines for Americans among adults aged 18 and over, by selected characteristics: United States, selected years 1998–2018. Hyattsville, MD; 2019. Available from: https://www.cdc.gov/nchs/hus/datafinder.htm.
2. Costello E, Leone JE, Ellzy M, Miller TA. Older adult perceptions of the physicians' role in promoting physical activity. Disabil Rehabil. 2013;35(14):1191–8.
3. Guralnik JM, Simonsick EM, Ferrucci L, Glynn RJ, Berkman LF, Blazer DG, et al. A short physical performance battery assessing lower extremity function: Association with self-reported disability and prediction of mortality and nursing home admission. J Gerontol. 1994;49(2):M85–94.
4. Rikli RE, Jones JJ. Functional fitness normative scores for community-residing older adults, 60-94. J Aging Phys Act. 1999;7:162–81.
5. Rikli RE, Jones CJ. Development and validation of a functoinal fitness test for community-residing older adults. J Aging Phys Act. 1999;7(2):129–61.
6. ATS Committee on Proficiency Standards for Clinical Pulmonary Function Laboratories. ATS statement: guidelines for the six-minute walk test. Am J Respir Crit Care Med. 2002;166:111–7.

7. Fritz S, Lusardi M. White paper: "walking speed: the sixth vital sign". J Geriatr Phys Ther. 2009;32(2):2–5.
8. Myers JN, Fonda H. The impact of fitness on surgical outcomes: the case for prehabilitation. Curr Sports Med Rep. 2016;15(4):282–9.
9. U.S. Department of Health and Human Services, editor. Physical activity guidelines for Americans. 2nd ed. Washington: U.S. Department of Health and Human Services; 2018.
10. Liguori G, Feito Y, Fountaine C, Roy BA, editors. ACSM's guidelines for exercise testing and prescription. 11th ed. Philadelphia: Wolters Kluwer; 2022.

Chapter 7
Social and Cultural Influences on Physical Activity

Madeleine E. Hackney and Tricia Creel

Key Points
- Understanding how individual, relationship, community, and society factors interact with older adults' understanding and access to exercise is key to promoting increased physical activity
- Underserved and historically minoritized older populations participate in recommended exercise typically less than other older adults, which is related to multiple barriers
- Studies considering these factors and barriers demonstrate successful strategies for older adults, for sustained exercise participation

Introduction

There are many acknowledged benefits of physical activity (PA), including reduced premature mortality, cardiovascular disease, hypertension, type 2 diabetes, and several types of cancers [1]. Beyond these health advantages, physical activity also contributes to improved cognition, weight management, fall risks, and ability to complete daily activities [2]. Despite these acknowledged benefits, in 2020 US adults over 65 had the lowest participation rates for strengthening and endurance activities [3]. Participation rates for adults were also lowest for communities of color and those with the lowest family incomes [3]. These individuals often

M. E. Hackney (✉)
Department of Medicine, Emory University School Medicine, Atlanta VA Health Care System, Center for Visual and Neurocognitive Rehabilitation, Atlanta, GA, USA
e-mail: mehackn@emory.edu

T. Creel
MDT Education Solutions, Atlanta, MO, USA

encounter complex, multi-factorial barriers, including institutional, social, cultural, and environmental difficulties [1].

To understand older adults' sedentary behaviors and how to promote physical activity in underserved populations, this chapter will use the socioecological model (SEM) to discuss facilitators and barriers to health-promoting behaviors, specifically, participation in physical activity. This chapter will discuss individual, relational, community, and public policy factors that influence an individual's ability to start and sustain an exercise program. In addition, this chapter will explore evidence-based interventions, culturally and linguistically tailored to meet the needs of specific populations, which increase physical activity in older adults. Finally, this chapter will provide questions for program evaluation, to understand effects of interventions from the older adult perspective.

The Socioecological Model

The SEM model describes how individual and population health are influenced by multilevel factors interacting to support or undermine a certain behavior [4]. This framework provides a method for evaluating the multiple layers of factors that can affect behavior; each layer contributes to the complete picture and each layer influences the next [5] (Fig. 7.1).

At the center of the model is the *individual*. This layer includes personal characteristics such as age, gender, education level, beliefs, life experiences, and attitudes, all of which influence the likelihood of an individual participating in physical activity. Interventions that target this layer of the model tend to focus on changing or increasing an individual's knowledge, outlook, skills, and abilities [5]. The next level is *relationships*, which describes an individual's familial and social networks that may influence their health-related practices and health decision-making. For example, having a physically active friend, colleague, or a family member can positively affect an individual's exercise behavior. Strategies that target this layer may include educating caregivers, programs that facilitate social interactions with peers, and mentoring.

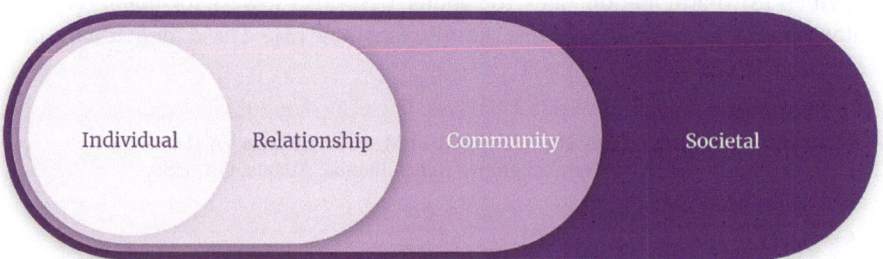

Fig. 7.1 Socioecological model which can be applied to older adults and physical activity. Graphic found at https://www.cdc.gov/violenceprevention/about/social-ecologicalmodel.html

The *community* level describes how local institutions and the environment, such as walking trails or affordable fitness centers, can shape participation in physical activity. In addition to individual and relational levels, it is important to acknowledge external contributions. The dynamics within a community play a role in healthy behavior participation and the perception of the benefits of engaging in an activity. For example, individuals may feel unsafe walking in their neighborhood or may feel that the marginal utility of investing in their health, such as through exercise, is reduced when the prospect of longevity is threatened by more immediate violence or poverty.

The final level of the SEM, *societal*, encompasses the rules, regulations, laws, and government policies that impact physical activity. Policies and funding—or lack of funding—can substantially affect access to appropriate physical environments for exercise and the adoption of behaviors favoring increased physical activity (Fig. 7.2).

A Socioecological Approach to Increasing Physical Activity in Older Adults

Individual: Accessible and affordable content/programs that address cultural, social, physical and cognitive function through positive engagement, leading to increased PA.

Relationships: Caregiver, peer, and familial involvement in social, fun, culturally appropriate physical activities that address psychosocial needs. Nurturing healthy relationships to facilitate sustainable changes in PA.

Community: Accessible, affordable exercise studios, gyms, and community spaces that allow diverse older adults to participate in PA; transportation to these areas and trained staff to support participants.

Societal: Local, state, and national laws fostering physical activity spaces and creative exercise approaches that make PA more accessible and appropriate for older individuals of diverse backgrounds.

PA = physical activity

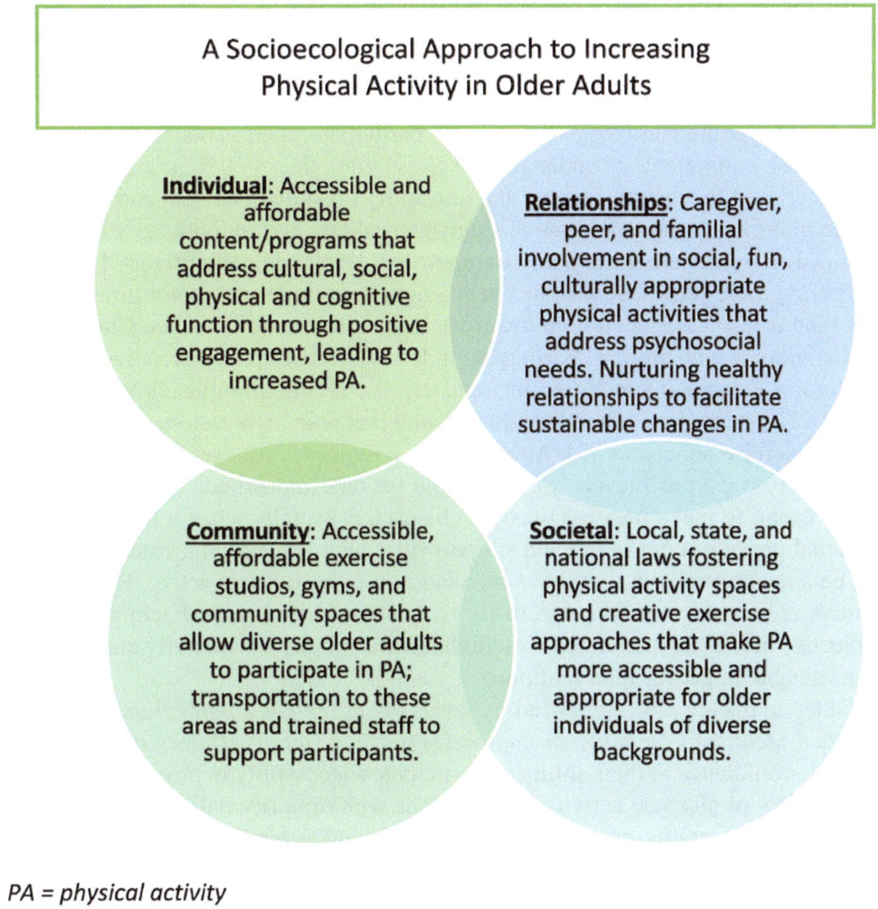

Fig. 7.2 Socioecological approaches to increasing physical activity in older adults

Individual Factors

Many older adults find it difficult to sustain an exercise program. Some of the common individual barriers are physical limitations, fear of falling, lack of motivation, not finding time, not knowing how to exercise, not understanding exercise benefits, adverse perceptions of exercise, and lack of self-efficacy. However, there are also individual facilitators that can be leveraged to promote exercise, including a previous history of exercise, absence of pain, and understanding the benefits of exercise.

Demographics, knowledge, education, and *gender* all factor into whether a person is physically active. For example, older women who are influenced by traditional gender roles may be more active in some domains, such as housework and childcare, while older men may pursue physical activity through leisure sports activities. These patterns may change as subsequent generations reach older adulthood. New research suggests that women may prefer fitness instruction provided in-person, not via smartphone apps, while men prefer using smartphone apps to complete guided exercise. Accounting for gender-based patterns in both the type of activity and delivery method may improve exercise participation in older adults [6]. Higher education levels are associated with higher physical activity levels particularly when specific knowledge is needed to participate, such as how to participate in a sport, use equipment, or understand exercise guidelines [7]. Research has shown a link between low health literacy and unhealthy lifestyle behaviors and that racial/ethnic minority groups, non-native English speakers, and individuals with limited financial resources are more likely to report low levels of health literacy [1].

Frailty, more prevalent with increasing age, is an important factor limiting exercise (and is also associated with lower socioeconomic status [8] (See Chaps. 1 and 2). Individuals who are frail participate in lower levels of physical activity, participate in fewer social interactions, and tend to present with multiple chronic diseases. In a 2021 systematic review the authors found that pain, depression, or fatigue may reduce exercise adherence [9]. Alternatively, a major health event can have a positive effect on exercise levels. Some people become motivated, by a diagnosis or health event, to make positive lifestyle changes, especially when a healthcare professional provides counseling and support [9]. Other research indicates that it may not be a health problem that prevents older adults from being active. Rather, what matters is how the person subjectively feels about their health. Feelings of better subjective health are associated with higher levels of physical activity and thus may be a valuable target for interventions.

Older adults are also influenced by levels of *self-efficacy, perception of benefits,* and their *identity as an active or non-active person* [7]. Self-efficacy is defined as a person's confidence in their ability to participate successfully in physical activity. A 2015 review of physical activity interventions with minority individuals found that interventions targeting either self-efficacy or social support reported the greatest changes in physical activity behaviors [10]. A 2017 systematic review showed that for older adults, higher levels of motivation and self-efficacy were associated with higher levels of physical activity [7]. Self-efficacy influences an individual's activity initiation and persistence, while a low level can be related to avoidance of the activity.

Older adults may also have negative beliefs about the consequences of exercise, including fear of falling, belief that they risk "overdoing it," or being unsure whether a certain exercise will be beneficial. Finally, the person's history of participation in exercise and their perception of themselves as being an active or non-active person can have a significant impact on their activity level, despite their actual health status. For example, Afshari et al. found that people with Parkinson's disease who were previously high exercisers were more likely to continue intense exercise after being diagnosed, versus low-exercisers who were more likely to reduce their participation in exercise [11].

It is also important to recognize how older individuals may respond behaviorally to increases in formal exercise. A 2018 study of 1020 adults who completed previous-day recalls of time spent in sedentary and physical activity showed that on days where participants completed formal exercise, they reported an average of 1.33 h/day of exercise, but this was often exchanged from other time use categories: they reported less sedentary time but also less light activity, household, work, and shopping activities on exercise days. The result was that on days where individuals participated in formal exercise, they often decreased energy expenditure from everyday activities [12]. Thus, interventions designed to increase total physical activity may need to include a holistic approach, to incorporate both formal exercise and daily life task activities, for an overall physical activity plan.

Relationship Factors

Social Networks, Engagement, Norms

In a 2021 systematic review of qualitative literature on factors influencing physical activity in community dwelling stroke survivors, the authors noted that the strongest influencers were *social networks* and *social engagement* [13]. Family members and friends can encourage physical activity when the individual is not motivated. Additionally, individuals are more likely to participate when their involvement is important to another person, they have an activity scheduled, or they perceive that someone is relying on their engagement. As one participant said:

> Sometimes I'm bad some days, I don't want to walk, I just think, oh, I've had enough. And then he'll say, come on let's go for our walk, and every time I do, I am always glad we did go. [14]

Social support, defined broadly as connections, assistance, or encouragement from family members, friends, co-workers, and community members, is a widely recognized social determinant of health. Higher levels of social support are strongly associated with higher levels of physical activity, specifically leisure activities [15]. Other interpersonal factors that have been shown to positively influence physical activity in older adults include: larger social networks; closer or reciprocated connections within the social network; similarity in physical activity pursuits between the person and their social network; being exposed to physical activity through their social network, which increases the sense of social norms relative to exercise; and connecting with others engaged in exercise who have similar demographic characteristics such as age, race, or sex [16].

Social norms are the cultural context within which a person's relationships are shaped. Older adults are influenced by the social norms within their social support networks. Often subjective and unwritten standards, these norms may influence behaviors in a particular direction. For example, the presence of others walking in the neighborhood can prompt activity in a previously inactive person. In a study of influences on physical activity in rural adults, one participant reported that seeing others being active prompted the thought, *"I could do that too"* [14].

Thus, it is important to adopt a holistic approach to understanding each cultural group. Practitioners should seek to understand any attitudes and beliefs that could hinder exercise participation, but also to recognize each cultural group's unique resources and strengths, which can be accessed to effectively promote engagement in exercise. Melillo et al. found a cultural sentiment among Hispanic/Latino respondents that exercise and physical activity are not appropriate for older adults and may lead to injury [17]. Bantham et al. observed cultural challenges for African American women, who reported perceptions that participation in physical activity is "selfish" and takes time away from caring for their family [1]. However, cultural groups may also have assets that can be leveraged to overcome obstacles to physical activity, including multi-generational living situations, connections to music, dance or specific sports, and a value system that promotes caring for elders.

Relationship with Healthcare Practitioners

Healthcare practitioners generally support physical activity for older adults. Clinicians typically prescribe exercise for older adults following guidelines from the American College of Sports Medicine, the Centers for Disease Control (CDC), and other groups. However, these recommendations alone are not sufficient to increase the number of older adults who exercise nor the frequency at which they exercise. For example, a study from 2022 showed that in the UK, although the chief medical officer strongly recommended strength training for all older adults two times per week, the vast majority of older adults surveyed had never heard of the recommendation and instead suggested non-targeted activities, e.g., walking, as suitable for increasing strength [18]. In fact, research shows that to enhance the clinician–patient relationship, older adults need adequate time to broach their own ideas about self-care actions, including lifestyle changes, with a practitioner who is willing to listen [19].

Relationships with Fitness Instructors and Personal Trainers

Older adults often will attend an exercise class or session when a strong relationship has been developed with the fitness instructor, personal trainer, or other type of physical activity coach. Studies have shown that it is important for instructors to develop rapport with participants in their session, support autonomous engagement, show care, foster trust through expert instruction, manage conflict directly and effectively, and create a climate where people want to be [20]. In addition to the mechanics of delivering a physical activity with clear cueing and safety instructions, instructor training should include understanding the social aspects of exercise delivery, and consider older adults' diverse needs and preferences for social interaction [21].

Community Factors

The community encompasses an older adult's neighborhood, senior living facility or residence, peer groups of all kinds, religious organizations, the larger group of extended family and friends, and any group or center that is considered proximal or local by an individual. Community has an outsize impact on whether an individual pursues physical activities: the older adult's identity can be strikingly attached to their community. The community often provides the most direct barriers and facilitators to participation, especially for group activities.

Environment. Several environmental factors may contribute to the suitability for older adults to engage in physical activity. Many researchers believe that outdoor mobility enables older adults' independence and social engagement within their community [22]. Davis et al. demonstrated that using public transportation or walking for transportation can lead to increased physical activity [23]. Research shows that older adult health outcomes, including those resulting from pursuit or nonpursuit of physical activity, are likely to be influenced by the neighborhood in which older adults live [24].

A walkable neighborhood with trees may encourage older adults to walk more [25]. Greenness of a neighborhood can be assessed by satellite, to quantify the amount of green vegetation within a certain distance of residences. A Canadian study showed that greenness may moderate the relationship between physical activity and mobility impairment in older adults [24].

Safety is another important consideration. Whether older adults find an area safe to walk in results from an intersection of individual perceptions and elements of the social environment, which is defined by immediate physical surroundings, social relationships and cultural backdrops [22]. Safely navigating sidewalks and crosswalks is imperative for older adults: sidewalks must exist and be maintained, and crosswalks need to provide ample time for crossing [26].

Air pollution in increasingly an issue for older adults who engage in outside exercise [27]. A 2023 systematic review found that, although air pollutants can adversely impact health in older adults, overall it is better to engage in physical activity than to continue sedentary behaviors [28]. Yet, both the level of air pollution and communications about air pollution may discourage older adults from engaging in outside exercise [29].

A safe, walkable neighborhood with destinations nearby, greenness, and relatively low levels of air pollution is likely to encourage more older adults to adopt physical activities. While the neighborhood is experienced at the community level by individuals, societal factors largely influence the state of one's neighborhood.

Cultural Influences

Culturally relevant exercise interventions will address the sociocultural, norms, societal expectations, and behaviors of the intended population. Different racial and ethnic groups have varying conceptions of "successful aging" and these concepts should affect exercise approaches [30, 31]. Providing culturally relevant activities can result in increased uptake and participation. For example, providing Latin dance classes may lead to enhanced participation and benefits to cognition and mobility in older adults [32]. Black women have increased mobility and physical activity through culturally appropriate and tailored interventions, such as a Prime Time Sister Circles program [33]. Lishi, a culturally-based, East Asian movement program, promoted greater self-efficacy, energy and balance and reduced pain in older Vietnamese adults enrolled in a randomized controlled trial [34].

Tango and Tai Chi are good examples of interventions that can cross cultures with widespread appeal. Tai Chi, derived from China and East Asia, is an exemplar of a culturally appropriate intervention that is now mainstream and widely recognized as a fall prevention exercise. Abundant research supports it and its corollaries, such as Qigong, for reducing falls in older adults. Latin dance, such as tango, could become just as widespread. It has been shown to be effective for improving balance, mobility, and cognition (Fig. 7.3). For example, older adults with Parkinson's and cognitive impairment may benefit from engaging in an adapted form of Argentine tango dance [35]. *Adaptango* has also been successfully tested as an intervention for middle to older aged African American women at risk for developing dementia [36, 37].

The key principles for improving uptake of physical activity by diverse racial and ethnic groups are using community health representatives to lead physical activity interventions and culturally adapting programs for a particular ethnic or racial group. These tenets are well described in an exercise trial for Zuni elders, who will experience a culturally adapted Otago Exercise program led by community members, to promote program sustainability. Such approaches are extremely important for remote areas whose residents do not have easy access to physical therapy, fitness personnel, or other health professionals [38].

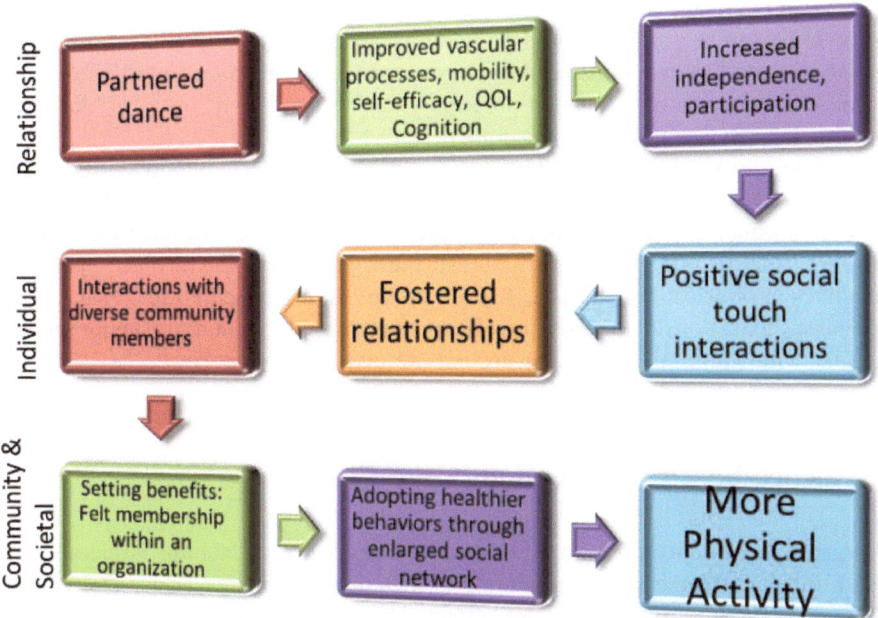

Fig. 7.3 The path to increased activity via partnered dance. The figure below shows one exemplar of physical activity, *Partnered Dance*, and the path through which the practice appears to lead to increased physical activity

Societal Factors

Society benefits from promoting physical activity to reduce overall healthcare use, as there is a negative association between physical activity and overnight hospitalization or home health care services, as well as the benefits to many health conditions [39]. Although engagement in physical activity depends on intrapersonal, relationship, cultural, community, and physical environment factors, it is society's decision-makers who determine investments in the built environment, to promote or dissuade mobility in older adults [22, 40]. Policy-makers influence whether older adults, regardless of income or background, have access to exercise. Societies use numerous strategies to promote greater or lesser physical activity in a population.

For example, a substantial portion of older adults have reduced vision, from age-related macular degeneration, glaucoma, and diabetes mellitus. Access for these individuals is promoted by inclusive—both built and social—environments and comprehensible information about physical activity benefits, and is reduced by fear and safety concerns, misinformation or lack of information, and unsupportive organizations [41]. Society can use this information as a blueprint for shaping an inclusive environment for physical activity in all older adults.

An example of an inclusive vision is the ENJOY Seniors Exercise Park program, a funded project which uses specialized outdoor equipment and physical activity programs to engage seniors in exercise. The program was cost-effective and under-scores the importance of shared community spaces for motivating seniors to be safely active [42]. Programs need not be expensive: low-resource, multimodal exercise, and behavior maintenance programs have been shown to help older adults retain physical function over year-long periods [43].

Another example of societal effects on activity in older adults occurred during the COVID-19 pandemic, in which inactivity greatly increased in older adults. Social distancing was recommended; while individuals could exercise at home using virtual or other means, the overall message to "shelter in place" produced declines in physical activity [42, 43]. While this policy appeared necessary, future policies should consider the serious effects of increased sedentary behavior on older adults, with additional messaging around exercise.

Evidence-Based Interventions

Targeted community programming is most effective for reaching vulnerable and traditionally underserved populations, to meaningfully increase physical activity. These groups are disproportionately affected by chronic diseases that would benefit from exercise participation. The goal is to move from "reactive, secondary prevention (i.e., initiating treatment after a chronic disease diagnosis has occurred and subsequently managing that condition for the remainder of an individual's life)… to proactive, with the goal being primary prevention (i.e., preventing a chronic disease diagnosis" [1].

Effective community programming requires thoughtful planning, collaboration, funding, and engagement of community members in a culturally and linguistically appropriate manner. Physical activity participation is a complex behavior and requires a layered approach, guided by the needs of the target community and population. This section highlights a few community programs and research interventions that have demonstrated success (Table 7.1).

Enhance®Fitness Research indicates that older Hispanic/Latino adults are less likely to engage in exercise than non-Hispanic/White older adults. In addition to decreased access to transportation and exercise facilities, cultural sentiments might contribute to lower physical activity levels. This includes the belief that older age inevitably coincides with declines in activity and mobility. A 2016 study looked at the effect of providing attribution retraining, in which older adults learned to view declines in health and mobility with aging as a controllable attribute that they could influence [44]. The retraining was provided in tandem with free Enhance®Fitness exercise classes at a senior center. Enhance®Fitness is an evidence-based program for seniors that is available in YMCAs, senior centers, churches, and recreation centers nationwide. The study found trends that suggested attribution retraining might have a positive impact on participants' long-term exer-

Table 7.1 Sample community programs and research interventions best practices

Community program	Location(s)	Target population	Key components
Enhance®Fitness and Enhance®Wellness	YMCAs, senior centers, churches, and recreation centers	Older adults	– Evidence-based – Low cost – Group exercise and falls prevention – Led by certified instructors – Participant progress tracked with fitness checks – Connects participants with a personal health and wellness coach
Restoring Balance	Homes and training sites in Arizona	Native Americans during and/or after cancer treatment	– Free, part of a research study – Designed with focus groups and interviews with community members and cultural experts – Employs Native trainers and staff – Holistic perspective – Trainer supervised exercise paired with home exercise program – Family inclusion encouraged
Walk With Ease	Communities, work places	Adults with arthritis, older adults, adults living in rural areas	– Evidence-based – Grants for group program, low cost to implement if self-directed – Program flexibility – Community partnerships – Program champions – Offers health education and motivational strategies
PAACE	YMCA and homes	African-American older adults, older adults	– Focus group input – Community-based marketing including in-person presentations at churches, sororities/fraternities, community centers, local media – Combination of home and group exercise – Free

cise participation. However, the study showed that access to an appropriate fitness program and social supports, such as coaches, was more important for behavior change [44].

Restoring Balance Another example of enhancing access to exercise programs is a physical activity program developed by the University of Arizona specifically for Native Americans who are cancer survivors. *Restoring Balance* follows American College of Sports Medicine Exercise Guidelines for Cancer Survivors, while also ensuring that interventions are aligned with traditional cultural preferences and participation is realistic [45]. The intervention used focus groups, interviews, and input from cultural experts to understand: (1) perspectives on physical activity; (2) motivators for physical activity; (3) barriers to physical activity; and (4) preference for delivery, type, and elements of physical activity programs. The program includes a hybrid of supervised exercise at a training facility and at-home exercise. This approach was important for participants in areas with infrastructure challenges. Other key components include encouragement of family supporters to join the exercise program with the participant and having Native trainers and staff delivering the intervention [45].

Walk with Ease The Arthritis Foundation's *Walk with Ease* program is a 6-week course that encourages participants to walk three times a week. It can be self-directed or done as a group with a volunteer leader. The program includes a low-cost workbook that provides lessons on health education, stretching and strengthening exercises, and motivational strategies. The program has shown benefits with diverse racial/ethnic groups. A 2022 study looked at five community-based organizations that received 1-year grants to implement the program [46]. The study evaluated implementation barriers and characteristics of successful versus unsuccessful organizations. Barriers identified included competition for physical space and staff time, difficulty engaging older adults, difficulty recruiting and retaining volunteer leaders, and the 3-day per week commitment. The study noted key factors for overcoming barriers: (1) where possible, use staff instead of volunteers to lead, (2) allow program flexibility to meet specific community needs, (3) partner with the community to recruit participants, (4) identify internal program champions [46].

PAACE The activity levels of many older African Americans are below recommended national guidelines. A 2022 intervention, the *Program for African American Cognition and Exercise*, looked at whether physical activity levels could be increased with a program designed with focus group input from older African Americans [47]. Participants were randomized to a successful aging group (SAG) or a physical activity group (PAG) for 12 weeks. The PAG included a combination of weekly group exercise sessions and home-based exercises. The SAG consisted of weekly group education sessions on aspects of healthy aging. The PAG group increased physical activity, with high group session attendance rates and high satisfaction. Participants were more active on days when they attended supervised group sessions but did not reach target activity levels on the 2–3 days/week for home-based activities. Study authors proposed that limiting factors included reduced accountability, difficulty assessing what entailed moderate-to-vigorous activity, lack of social support, and lack of understanding of behavior change strategies. This is an important future research area as not all older adults have access or want to participate in supervised group exercise programs [47].

Conclusion

Underserved groups often face unique barriers to participation in regular physical activity. These barriers can exist at all levels of the socioecological model, including individual, interpersonal, community, environmental, and societal. As a result, effective interventions need to be collaborative efforts that are informed by and tailored to the needs of the specific population. This collaboration may include community members, healthcare professionals, public health professionals, policymakers, researchers, and the business community. As shown in the highlighted programs, effective programs are culturally and linguistically specific, take place in accessible and welcoming locations, are affordable and flexible, include an education component, engage family member support, are led by trusted community members, and provide accountability. To understand program fit with older adults' needs and interests as these evolve, ongoing program evaluation will be essential (Table 7.2).

Table 7.2 Sample questions for evaluating older adults' exercise program experiences

Individual	– Tell us about your physical activity since participating in the intervention. Have you been able to do the things you want to do? – What sorts of physical activities have you been engaged in outside of the intervention, since it began? – How have you felt mentally since coming here? – Are these physical or mental activities different or similar to ones you did before the intervention? *Probe for factors associated with change or lack of change in physical or mental activities* – What is the most important thing you have gotten out of this program? Was there anything that was not helpful?
Relationship	– Tell us about your experience in the program with your care partner/friend/loved one. What was it like participating in the program with your care partner? What has your experience been like with other people here? *Probe for positive or negative experiences and factors associated with these experiences* – What have your relationships been like with close friends, and family since starting the program? Has anything changed? – Thinking about the things you and your care partner need to do in your daily lives, did the class schedule work for you? *Probe for factors associated with why the approach was perceived as working for their schedules or not*
Community	– Tell me about your relationships with your community, with this space and the people who work out here? How do the people involved at this place make you feel? – Has anything changed in your community since participating in the intervention? Has coming to this space impacted the groups that you go around with? – What did you think of places to exercise before the intervention? Has your attitude changed? How has your experience at this community space affected what you do on a daily basis and the kinds of activities you do?
Societal	– Tell me how you feel about society's attitudes towards you adding physical activity into your life. What do you think society expects from someone like you in regards to physical activity? – How does society support physical activity for people in your peer group? – How does society prevent or hinder your peer group from achieving physical activity? – Does society value physical activity? For you? For your peer group? For your family members? – How have your perceptions of society in relation to physical activity impacted what you do on a daily basis? Over the years?

References

1. Bantham A, Ross SET, Sebastião E, Hall G. Overcoming barriers to physical activity in underserved populations. Prog Cardiovasc Dis. 2021;64:64–71.
2. CDC. Benefits of physical activity. 2023. https://www.cdc.gov/physicalactivity/basics/pa-health/index.htm. Accessed 24 July 2023.
3. CDC WEB. https://www.cdc.gov/nchs/products/databriefs/db443.htm. Accessed 24 July 2023.
4. Olaniyan A, Isiguzo C, Hawk M. The Socioecological Model as a framework for exploring factors influencing childhood immunization uptake in Lagos state, Nigeria. BMC Public Health. 2021;21(1):867.

5. Tehrani H, Majlessi F, Shojaeizadeh D, Sadeghi R, Kabootarkhani MH. Applying socioeco-logical model to improve women's physical activity: a randomized control trial. Iran Red Crescent Med J. 2016;18(3):e21072.
6. Lee YL, Lee GS, Teo LL, Tan R-S, Zhong L, Gao F, Koh AS. Effect of psychosocial motivations and technology on physical activity behaviours among community older men and women. BMC Geriatr. 2022;22(1):933.
7. Notthoff N, Reisch P, Gerstorf D. Individual characteristics and physical activity in older adults: a systematic review. Gerontology. 2017;63(5):443–59.
8. McPhee JS, French DP, Jackson D, Nazroo J, Pendleton N, Degens H. Physical activity in older age: perspectives for healthy ageing and frailty. Biogerontology. 2016;17:567–80.
9. Collado-Mateo D, Lavín-Pérez AM, Peñacoba C, Del Coso J, Leyton-Román M, Luque-Casado A, Gasque P, Fernández-del-Olmo MÁ, Amado-Alonso D. Key factors associated with adherence to physical exercise in patients with chronic diseases and older adults: an umbrella review. Int J Environ Res Public Health. 2021;18(4):2023.
10. Mama SK, McNeill LH, McCurdy SA, Evans AE, Diamond PM, Adamus-Leach HJ, Lee RE. Psychosocial factors and theory in physical activity studies in minorities. Am J Health Behav. 2015;39(1):68–76.
11. Afshari M, Yang A, Bega D. Motivators and barriers to exercise in Parkinson's disease. J Parkinsons Dis. 2017;7(4):703–11.
12. Matthews CE, Keadle SK, Saint-Maurice PF, Moore SC, Willis EA, Sampson JN, Berrigan D. Use of time and energy on exercise, prolonged TV viewing, and work days. Am J Prev Med. 2018;55(3):e61–9.
13. Espernberger KR, Fini NA, Peiris CL. Personal and social factors that influence physical activity levels in community-dwelling stroke survivors: a systematic review of qualitative literature. Clin Rehabil. 2021;35(7):1044–55.
14. Kubina L-A, Dubouloz C-J, Davis CG, Kessler D, Egan MY. The process of re-engagement in personally valued activities during the two years following stroke. Disabil Rehabil. 2013;35(3):236–43.
15. Amorim TC, Azevedo MR, Hallal PC. Physical activity levels according to physical and social environmental factors in a sample of adults living in South Brazil. J Phys Act Health. 2010;7(2):S204–12.
16. Prochnow T, Patterson MS. Assessing social network influences on adult physical activity using social network analysis: a systematic review. Am J Health Promot. 2022;36(3):537–58.
17. Melillo KD, Williamson E, Houde SC, Futrell M, Read CY, Campasano M. Perceptions of older Latino adults regarding physical fitness, physical activity, and exercise. SLACK Incorp Thorofare. 2001;27:38–46.
18. Gluchowski A, Bilsborough H, Mcdermott J, Hawley-Hague H, Todd C. 'A lot of people just go for walks, and don't do anything else': older adults in the UK are not aware of the strength component embedded in the chief medical officers' physical activity guidelines—a qualitative study. Int J Environ Res Public Health. 2022;19(16):10002.
19. Rees S, Williams A. Promoting and supporting self-management for adults living in the community with physical chronic illness: a systematic review of the effectiveness and meaningfulness of the patient-practitioner encounter. JBI Evid Synth. 2009;7(13):492–582.
20. Morrison L, McDonough MH, Zimmer C, Din C, Hewson J, Toohey A, Crocker PR, Bennett EV. Instructor social support in the group physical activity context: older participants' perspectives. J Aging Phys Act. 2023;1:1–11.
21. Zimmer C, McDonough MH, Hewson J, Toohey A, Din C, Crocker PR, Bennett EV. Experiences with Social Participation in group physical activity programs for older adults. J Sport Exerc Psychol. 2021;43(4):335–44.
22. Hanson HM, Schiller C, Winters M, Sims-Gould J, Clarke P, Curran E, Donaldson MG, Pitman B, Scott V, McKay HA. Concept mapping applied to the intersection between older adults' outdoor walking and the built and social environments. Prev Med. 2013;57(6):785–91.

23. Davis MG, Fox KR, Hillsdon M, Coulson JC, Sharp DJ, Stathi A, Thompson JL. Getting out and about in older adults: the nature of daily trips and their association with objectively assessed physical activity. Int J Behav Nutr Phys Act. 2011;8:1–9.
24. Putman A, Klicnik I, Dogra S. Neighbourhood greenness moderates the association between physical activity and geriatric-relevant health outcomes: an analysis of the CLSA. BMC Geriatr. 2023;23(1):317.
25. Klicnik I, Cullen JD, Doiron D, Barakat C, Ardern CI, Rudoler D, Dogra S. Leisure sedentary time and physical activity are higher in neighbourhoods with denser greenness and better built environments: an analysis of the Canadian Longitudinal Study on Aging. Appl Physiol Nutr Metab. 2022;47(3):278–86.
26. Corseuil MW, Schneider IJC, Silva DAS, Costa FF, Silva KS, Borges LJ, d'Orsi E. Perception of environmental obstacles to commuting physical activity in Brazilian elderly. Prev Med. 2011;53(4-5):289–92.
27. Roberts JD, Voss JD, Knight B. The association of ambient air pollution and physical inactivity in the United States. PLoS One. 2014;9(3):e90143.
28. D'Oliveira A, Dominski FH, De Souza LC, Branco JHL, Matte DL, da Cruz WM, Andrade A. Impact of air pollution on the health of the older adults during physical activity and sedentary behavior: a systematic review. Environ Res. 2023;2023:116519.
29. An R, Shen J, Ying B, Tainio M, Andersen ZJ, de Nazelle A. Impact of ambient air pollution on physical activity and sedentary behavior in China: a systematic review. Environ Res. 2019;176:108545.
30. Reich AJ, Claunch KD, Verdeja MA, Dungan MT, Anderson S, Clayton CK, Goates MC, Thacker EL. What does "successful aging" mean to you? Systematic review and cross-cultural comparison of lay perspectives of older adults in 13 countries, 2010–2020. J Cross Cult Gerontol. 2020;35:455–78.
31. Resnicow K, Baranowski T, Ahluwalia JS, Braithwaite RL. Cultural sensitivity in public health: defined and demystified. Ethn Dis. 1999;9(1):10–21.
32. Aguiñaga A, Kaushal N, Balbim GM, Wilson RS, Wilbur JE, Hughes S, et al. Latin dance and working memory: the mediating effects of physical activity among middle-aged and older Latinos. Front Aging Neurosci. 2022;14:755154.
33. Ibe CA, Haywood DR, Creighton C, Cao Y, Gabriel A, Zare H, Jones W, Yang M, Balamani M, Gaston M. Study protocol of a randomized controlled trial evaluating the Prime Time Sister Circles (PTSC) program's impact on hypertension among midlife African American women. BMC Public Health. 2021;21:1–10.
34. Huang CY, Zane NW, Hunter L, Vang L, Apesoa-Varano EC, Joseph J. Promoting mental and physical health of Vietnamese immigrants through a cultural movement intervention. Cultur Divers Ethnic Minor Psychol. 2023. https://doi.org/10.1037/cdp0000591.
35. Hackney ME, Bay AA, Jackson JM, Nocera JR, Krishnamurthy V, Crosson B, Evatt ML, Langley J, Cui X, McKay JL. Rationale and design of the PAIRED trial: partnered dance aerobic exercise as a neuroprotective, motor, and cognitive intervention in Parkinson's Disease. Front Neurol. 2020;11:943.
36. Wharton W, Jeong L, Ni L, Bay AA, Shin RJ, McCullough LE, Silverstein H, Hart AR, Swieboda D, Hu W. A pilot randomized clinical trial of adapted tango to improve cognition and psychosocial function in African American women with family history of Alzheimer's disease (ACT trial). Cereb Circ Cogn Behav. 2021;2:100018.
37. Cao K, Bay AA, Hajjar I, Wharton W, Goldstein F, Qiu D, Prusin T, McKay JL, Perkins MM, Hackney ME. Rationale and design of the PARTNER trial: partnered rhythmic rehabilitation for enhanced motor-cognition in prodromal Alzheimer's disease. J Alzheimers Dis. 2023;91(3):1019–33.
38. Waters DL, Popp J, Herman C, Ghahate D, Bobelu J, Pankratz VS, Shah VO. The Otago Exercise Program compared to falls prevention education in Zuni elders: a randomized controlled trial. BMC Geriatr. 2022;22(1):1–12.

39. Jemna D-V, David M, Depret M-H, Ancelot L. Physical activity and healthcare utilization in France: evidence from the European Health Interview Survey (EHIS) 2014. BMC Public Health. 2022;22(1):1–20.
40. da Silva AS, Melo JCDN, Pereira ZS, Santos JCD, Silva RJDS, Araújo RHDO, Sampaio RAC. Correlates of physical activity in Brazilian older adults: the National Health Survey 2019. Int J Environ Res Public Health. 2023;20(3):2463.
41. Phoenix C, Griffin M, Smith B. Physical activity among older people with sight loss: a qualitative research study to inform policy and practice. Public Health. 2015;129(2):124–30.
42. Brusco NK, Hill KD, Haines T, Dunn J, Panisset MG, Dow B, Batchelor F, Biddle SJ, Duque G, Levinger P. Cost-effectiveness of the ENJOY seniors exercise park for older people: a pre–post intervention study. J Phys Act Health. 2023;20(6):555–65.
43. Stathi A, Withall J, Greaves CJ, Thompson JL, Taylor G, Medina-Lara A, Green C, Snowsill T, Johansen-Berg H, Bilzon J. A group-based exercise and behavioural maintenance intervention for adults over 65 years with mobility limitations: the REACT RCT. Southampton: National Institute for Health and Care Research; 2022.
44. Feldman JF, Hoyle MN. Isolation of circadian clock mutants of Neurospora crassa. Genetics. 1973;75(4):605–13.
45. Bea JW, Lane T, Charley B, Yazzie E, Yellowhair J, Hudson J, Kinslow B, Wertheim BC, Roe DJ, Schwartz A. Restoring balance: a physical activity intervention for native American cancer survivors and their familial support persons. Exerc Sport Movement. 2023;1(2):e00007.
46. Vilen LH, Altpeter M, Callahan LF. Overcoming barriers to walk with ease implementation in community organizations. Health Promot Pract. 2022;23(4):708–17.
47. Newton RL, Beyl R, Hebert C, Harris M, Carter L, Gahan W, Carmichael O. A physical activity intervention in older African Americans: the PAACE pilot randomized controlled trial. Med Sci Sports Exerc. 2022;54(10):1625–34.

Chapter 8
Exercise for Adults in Nursing Home and Assisted Living Facilities

Barbara Resnick

Key Points
- Older adults in skilled nursing, assisted living, and other short and long stay institutional settings benefit from participation in effective exercise programs
- Exercise is safe, although modifications are necessary, for institutionalized older adults
- Innovative strategies can motivate and engage older adults with different conditions and diseases, to participate in physical activities in institutional settings
- Both group and individual approaches can be used
- Residents living with dementia also benefit, cognitively and physically, from exercise
- Transforming the philosophy of care to include exercise is possible in institutional settings
- All members of the health care team need to support, encourage, and facilitate exercise activities among residents

Introduction

Despite known efficacy for improving function and health outcomes in older adults, in many if not most institutional settings the majority of provided activities do not include exercise or engagement in physical activities. Exercise, which is a subset of

Supplementary Information The online version contains supplementary material available at https://doi.org/10.1007/978-3-031-52928-3_8.

B. Resnick (✉)
Organizational Systems and Adult Health, School of Nursing, University of Maryland, Baltimore, MD, USA
e-mail: Resnick@umaryland.edu

© The Author(s), under exclusive license to Springer Nature Switzerland AG 2024
G. M. Sullivan, A. K. Pomidor (eds.), *Exercise for Aging Adults*,
https://doi.org/10.1007/978-3-031-52928-3_8

all physical activity, is defined by the American College of Sports Medicine as planned, structured, and repetitive bodily movements done to improve or maintain one or more physical fitness components. For most adults in institutional settings, the intensity and types of exercise will need to be modified. For example, aerobic conditioning requires that the intensity of the activity should range between 40 and 85% of aerobic capacity. For older adults in group settings, cardiorespiratory endurance often can be improved by conditioning at an intensity level as low as 40% of aerobic capacity or as few as 3000 steps/day. Moderate intensity aerobic exercise is experienced subjectively as little or no discomfort with a small increase in breathing rate. For the average adult, moderate intensity aerobic activity occurs when walking 100 steps in a minute. For older adults in institutional settings with multiple comorbid conditions, moderate aerobic activity may occur while walking to the bathroom. Thus, exercise for older adults can be subjectively defined by the individual: if it feels like exercise, then it is exercise.

In long-term care facilities, specifically nursing homes and assisted living communities, it has been repeatedly shown that increasing residents' participation in any type of exercise, at even low levels of intensity, results in improved gait, balance, and mood, and fewer disruptive behaviors. In addition, residents that optimize their function and physical activity are less likely to be transferred to the emergency room for episodes of care associated with non-fall-related problems, such as infections. Thus, there is substantial support to encourage older individuals in institutional settings to spend more time engaged in physical activity and less time in bed or sitting [1–3].

Despite the evidence supporting exercise in these settings, a persistent cycle may occur: deconditioning—existing prior to hospitalization or as a consequence of hospitalization—decreased function, contractures, and wheelchair dependence. After a resident has completed relevant rehabilitation services from physical and/or occupation therapy, often subsequent efforts to engage the resident in exercise is left to nursing staff, certified nursing assistants, direct care workers, and activity staff.

Case: Part 1

Beryl is an 80-year-old woman admitted to a long-term care facility for skilled rehabilitation after a hospital admission for fever, delirium, and influenza pneumonia. Previously, she lived alone in her own apartment with assistance for personal care activities from a private nursing assistant. At home she was able to ambulate 100 feet in the apartment; beyond that point, she would stop due to fatigue. Beryl has been treated for several years for Parkinson's disease, mild dementia, diabetes, hypertension, and depression. Beryl recovered slowly in the hospital; she first walked in her room with assistance on the fourth and final day. In the nursing facility she received physical and occupational therapy for several weeks. She made slow progress, was fearful of standing and resisted ambulating, and therapy was discontinued. Now, Beryl is in a wheelchair most of the day.

Exercise for Older Institutionalized Adults

The prevention of functional decline, which affects caregiving needs and quality of life, is critical for residents in long-term care. Being able to transfer with no or minimal assistance can facilitate a resident's ability to independently move about her room or within the facility. It may also allow a resident to get outside in a garden area, or visit a restaurant or family event. Furthermore, prevention of contractures, which often occur from sitting for long periods of time, will reduce future pain. Engaging in even limited exercise activities, such as doing sit-to-stand exercises (Box 8.1) and other simple activities that can be incorporated into daily activity [4], can greatly facilitate maintenance of function.

> **Box 8.1 Chair Sit-to-Stand**
> Start in a regular chair, sitting with your buttocks on the edge of the chair and your feet flat on the floor.
> Lean forward—nose over toes.
> Push with your legs and push your buttocks up. At the same time push down on the chair arms with your arms as counter leverage.
> To sit down, bend at your hips and reach back with your buttocks leading the way.
> Sit down slowly—do not drop down or fall backwards.
> *Start this at first by using your arms to help push you up, but work towards the goal of doing this without using your hands or arms.*

Aerobic, or endurance, training promotes optimal cardiovascular status by maintaining lung function and cardiac output. Strength training offsets the loss in muscle mass and strength that are commonly seen with aging and aggravated by disuse. Additional benefits from exercise include improved bone health, postural stability, and flexibility and range of motion (critical for bathing and dressing), and reduced fall risk and pain from stiff joints. Most important, exercise gives institutionalized older adults an overall sense of psychological health and well-being [5, 6]. Conversely, sedentary behavior and lack of activity promote deconditioning, contractures, pain, pressure ulcers, falls, and exacerbations of chronic illnesses.

Risks and Benefits of Exercise

Although studies show that the benefits of regular exercise for institutionalized older adults are greater than the risks, institutionalized older adults are more likely to have both cardiovascular and musculoskeletal conditions that warrant exercise modifications and enhanced awareness on the part of staff. Despite a higher prevalence of cardiovascular conditions, institutionalized older adults do not require additional screening before engaging in moderate levels of exercise, beyond the admission history, physical examination, and usual assessments. In fact, there is a greater risk of exacerbating and worsening cardiovascular disease from *not* exercising. However, those at greatest risk for cardiovascular events are individuals who previously were sedentary. To minimize the risk of cardiovascular events, it is essential that previously sedentary individuals, which will include many individuals in group settings, begin with low-rather than moderate-intensity exercise and increase slowly. As noted, a subjective appraisal of what is moderate activity can be used to establish exercise intensity for most older adults. The rating of perceived exertion (RPE) scale (see Chap. 4, Table 4.4) is a practical, easy method. The individual is asked to rate, on a scale of 1 (at rest exertion) to 10 (maximal exertion), how they perceive their exercise activity. For older adults with cognitive impairment, caregivers should ask how hard the older adult thinks they are working verbally rather than ask them to assign a number to the level of intensity. An RPE score that falls between 4 and 5 correlates with reaching 60–80% of the targeted heart rate or a moderate intensity of exercise.

Using good clinical judgment during exercise is critical for ensuring safety among older institutionalized adults. Table 8.1 lists the signs and symptoms staff should recognize and teach residents to be aware of and report, as potential danger signs during exercise. When these warning signs occur, exercise should be stopped and follow-up by the individual's health care clinician arranged.

Falls are the greatest risk that staff and residents fear, in association with exercise. While there is no evidence to support this fear, staff often encourage sedentary activities over exercise. Thus, for institutionalized older adults, it is particularly important to teach staff how to incorporate exercise activities that do not increase fall risks. For example, safe exercise equipment that individuals are not likely to fall off or trip over should be available. Appropriate supervision will be needed for individuals who have balance impairment. Staff will also need to monitor individuals with cognitive impairment who may have less awareness of their functional abilities or who must adhere to a specific weight-bearing status.

In comparison with cardiovascular events, musculoskeletal complaints and injuries are more likely to occur in older institutionalized adults. In general, older adults experience fewer musculoskeletal complications when exercising than younger

Table 8.1 Warning signs for nursing assistants, activity staff, families, and residents to recognize during exercise

Pale, clammy, cool skin
Change in cognition, such as new confusion or disorientation
Nausea or vomiting
Shortness of breath that does not resolve in 30 min
Chest pain
Dizziness
Unusual fatigue
Change in balance or unsteadiness

individuals, although deconditioning may predispose to increased risk. Fortunately, these complications are generally minor and often can be prevented. In order to decrease the risk of injury, "starting low and going slow" is highly recommended [7]. Likewise, monitoring for symptoms such as joint or muscle pain is critical, particularly for individuals with known joint conditions. Working up to but not to the point of pain, followed by rest, is advised. The majority of older adults, even those with cognitive impairment, are aware of discomfort or pain and will usually stop at this point. Some individuals may push beyond pain and require monitoring and counseling. Important parameters to monitor are evidence of pain; incorrect positioning, which can cause trauma; and working beyond one's capability, such as inability to talk while exercising.

Obese individuals and those with underlying arthritis, particularly in weight-bearing joints, will tolerate low-impact exercise such as pool-based exercises, stationary cycling, or walking better than high-impact activities. Starting with activities that do not cause pain or injury and building up slowly will facilitate adherence as well as prevent injuries. Exercise should be avoided in acutely inflamed or injured joints, until pain has substantially resolved.

Environmental Safety Considerations

The physical environment and appropriate exercise equipment are important aspects of safe exercising for institutionalized older adults. Age-appropriate equipment ensures that the individual is able to use the equipment correctly and safely. Table 8.2 provides an overview of considerations when selecting equipment for older adults. There are a growing number of continuing care retirement communities and larger long-term care settings that have exercise rooms housing age-appropriate devices. In addition, more facilities are including pools that allow for low-impact activities. A major advantage of institutional settings is that they provide open, flat, and clutter-free hallways with rails, for individuals to walk safely. The distances of facility hallways are often greater than those of the resident's prior home and thus can be used to significantly augment the amount of physical activity done by older institutional adults.

Weather, temperature, lighting, furniture, and clear open space influence exercise safety. Older adults are less able to adapt to heat and thus at risk for heat stress. During exercise, large amounts of heat are generated by active muscles. When it is hot and humid outside or when the inside environment is kept excessively warm, an older individual is less able to dissipate this heat. Unfortunately, older adults are both at greater risk for heat exhaustion and less likely to note prodromal symptoms. These symptoms include progressive weakness, fatigue, frontal headache, hypotension, tachycardia, and changes in cognition. Treatment of heat exhaustion requires cessation of exercise and rehydration. Obese individuals with multiple chronic illnesses and on multiple medications are particularly at risk for heat-related injuries. To reduce this risk, staff in institutional settings should determine when outdoor

Table 8.2 Safe exercise equipment for older adults

Key features	
Strength training equipment	User-friendly with nonintimidating appearance and function
	Lowest possible load or impact is available
	Non-obstructed entry and exit suitable for individuals with functional challenges or disability
	Clear, large-print instructions with diagrams
	Adjustable to various body sizes
	Able to change resistance levels when in a seated position
	Resistance levels that start low (less than 5 pounds) and increase at low increments such as 1 pound or less
	Range of motion adjustments that accommodate joint dysfunction or limitations due to joint replacements
	Easy adjustments to level of resistance for older adults with arthritis or stroke
Treadmills	Display panels with large buttons and letters that are easy to read
	Simple adjustment features that are easy for older adults to understand (e.g., up and down arrows to increase speed)
	Low starting speeds (e.g., 0.5 miles/h)
	Clear, large-print instructions with diagrams
	Shock-absorbing decks
	Emergency backup with belt clip so that the treadmill shuts off automatically if the individual stops moving or falls
	Low motor housing so it is possible to view the older individual while on the treadmill
	Handrails, for those with balance problems
Steppers, recumbent bikes	Open shroud entrance and exit
	Control panel that is easily accessible and easy to read
	Minimal preprogrammed workouts
	Clear, accessible adjustment features for seats and armrests that are within easy reach while seated
	Wide and comfortable seats with arm rests
	Swivel seats for easy entrance and exit

activity is safe and ensure that older residents wear loose clothing and maintain adequate hydration before and after exercising. Staff should avoid scheduling exercise activities in excessively warm or humid outside or inside conditions.

Environments that promote physical activity can reduce functional decline and enable people to achieve their highest level of function and well-being [8–10]. Designated exercise space may be limited or inaccessible in institutional settings. Hallways, common areas, and outdoor walkways are often available, yet seldom promoted for physical activity. Planning of institutional environments often focuses on safety rather than facilitating exercise and function. Case studies and direct observations of residential communities for older adults indicate that visibility of exercise-related areas, walkable spaces, clear open pathways, chairs that are the appropriate height for safe transferring by residents, and interesting walking destinations enhance exercise participation. Simple, cost-efficient modifications can improve exercise spaces, such as improved lighting, signs that specifically promote active living, and physical activity stations provided throughout the facility. Outdoor improvements include ensuring that sidewalks and stairs are safe and accessible, providing greenery and interesting destinations, and assuring adequate shade and seating so residents will feel comfortable outdoors.

In addition to consideration of the objective physical environment, the degree of *person-environment fit* (P-E fit) is critical to evaluate, especially as function declines. Adaptation, or P-E fit, occurs when there is a match between the person and the environment. Evidence suggests that individuals with lower function are particularly influenced by the P-E fit as they have to spend more energy overcoming and adapting to environments, and consequently are unable to optimally engage in physical activity. In these instances, physical activity can be improved by lowering environmental demands through interventions such as altering the height of a bed or a chair to facilitate transfers.

The height of a bed is critical for safety and to facilitate independent transfers. A bed that is too low is difficult to rise from. Conversely, a bed that is too high is difficult to get back on and lift the legs up on. The firmness of the mattress will also make a difference. An old mattress or one that "gives" under body weight is difficult to get onto and provides no support when pushing up to stand. Seat height should not be greater than 120% of lower leg length (LLL) or less that 80% of LLL as this can impede safe transfer and cause falls. Measurement of LLL is done from the kneecap to the ankle. Caregivers may resist changes in bed height, as the optimum height for caregivers who are helping with personal care or nursing activities and the best height to optimize transfer ability of the older adult are usually different. Height-adjustable beds and chairs are ideal in group settings. Height-adjustable beds are also useful if one height is needed for getting out of bed and another for getting into it.

Exercise Prescriptions for Institutionalized Adults

Individual Approaches

Health care providers are particularly challenged to determine what type and how much exercise to prescribe for older adults in institutional settings, where individual variation is the rule and deconditioning is rampant. While there are excellent resources for exercise activities for older adults, such as from the National Institute on Aging and Exercise is Medicine (see Resources), these exercise activities cannot generally be done independently by residents in long-term care settings. An effective method to engage older institutionalized adults in exercise activities is to incorporate exercise into daily life and activities, such as by adopting a *function-focused care* approach. Function-focused care is a philosophy of care that first evaluates the older adult's underlying capability with regard to function and physical activity [11, 12]. Then a plan is created to maintain abilities and continually increase time spent in physical activities. This philosophy of care is in contrast to routine long-term care approaches in which daily tasks are done by caregivers to ensure the individual is safe, well groomed, and dressed. Examples of function-focused care interactions include verbal cues during bathing so that the older individual performs the tasks rather than the direct care worker bathing the individual; asking the resident to walk to the bathroom rather than use a urinal; accompanying a resident to an exercise class; and initiating a few minutes of dancing.

Incorporating a function-focused care approach for an institutionalized older adult requires an individualized assessment. This is in contrast to assuming that the person is unable to perform a given activity (bathing, dressing, transferring), an exercise class will be too tiring or dangerous, or it will be easier to move the individual to the dining room or bathroom using a wheelchair. The focus should be on the task, not on getting the task completed. For example, in contrast to getting the resident to the dining room as quickly as possible, the task is having him or her walk during the move to the dining area. Focusing on task completion, rather than engagement of the resident in the task, propagates deconditioning and disability. Conversely, individuals need to be evaluated to determine if they have an underlying capability to perform the task: independently, with the assistance of another individual, or at the lowest level with hand-over-hand assistance (the caregiver performs the activity but moves the individual's arms through the motions, such as in eating). This determination will allow caregivers to establish appropriate exercise or physical activity goals.

The *Physical Capability Assessment* form is a straightforward method to identify the basic abilities of an older institutionalized resident and a critical first step to developing exercise goals. The basic elements of the physical capability assessment are shown in Table 8.3 and consist of simple functional tasks: one-, two-, or three-step commands; upper and lower extremity range of motion; transfers and ability to bear weight on lower extremities; and standing balance. Based on this assessment, and input from other members of the health care team, both functional and physical activity goals should be developed (Table 8.4). For example, if the individual has full range of motion and is able to follow at least a one-step command, he or she should be performing bathing and dressing with verbal cues as needed.

Case: Part 2

After Beryl was discharged from therapy, she remained at the nursing home, as she now needed 24-h personal assistance. Beryl scored 7 out of 16 on the Physical Capability Assessment. She had decreased range of motion in her upper extremities bilaterally. In the lower extremities, she had full range of motion at the ankle and knee and was able to march in place when sitting. She could not independently come to stand. With the assistance of one individual and verbal cues, she could come to stand and stand for 1 min. She was able to follow a single one-step command both verbally and visually. With this information, a specific exercise program and goals were established and incorporated into her care plan.

As Beryl could come to a stand with assistance, her first goal was to do three sit-to-stand exercises with every toilet transfer, or at least three times a

Table 8.3 Elements of the physical capability scale

Element	Test	Points
Range of motion	Upper extremity	
	Shoulder abduction	0–1
	Shoulder external	0–1
	Shoulder internal	0–1
	Lower extremity	
	Ankle flexion	0–1
	Ankle extension	0–1
	Knee	0–1
March while seated		0–1
Chair rise (chair sit-to-stand)	Stand from seated position	0–3
Follows commands	Single-step verbal	0–1
	Double-step verbal	0–1
	Triple-step verbal	0–1
	Single-step visual	0–1
	Double-step visual	0–1
	Triple-step visual	0–1
Total possible		16 (=highest function)

Adapted from Resnick et al. [13]

Table 8.4 Goal attainment scale guide

Patient name: _____				
Goal setter(s): _____				
Goal-setting date: _____ Follow-up date: _____ Goal attainment score (range −2 to +2; expected 0)				
Level of predicted attainment	Goal 1	Goal 2	Goal 3	Goal 4
Much less than expected −2				
Somewhat less than expected −1				
Expected 0				
Somewhat more than expected +1				
Much more than expected +2				

day. This was increased to do five sit-to-stand exercises (Box 8.1), after she could tolerate three. The goal form was reevaluated monthly. With time, she was able to stand for longer periods and ambulate short distances. Her next goals were walking three times a day, for a distance of approximately 20 feet, and chair-based group exercise activities offered in the facility.

Group Activities

Despite the benefits to engaging institutionalized older adults in exercise, initiating and continuing daily exercise programs remain an enormous challenge. Unfortunately, without continuing to offer and engage residents in exercise programs, deconditioning occurs [1]. There are many ways to incorporate group exercise into institutional settings that are low cost and appropriate for all residents. Examples of free resources are available (see Resources). Ten-minute spurts of exercise, done three times a day, can help residents and staff attain the minimum recommendations for physical activity for all adults [14, 15]. Dance is a terrific way to incorporate group exercise. Set aside 10-min periods for putting on fun dance tunes consistent with the cultural preferences of the residents and dance away to the music. Generally three to four songs will achieve the goal of 10 min. To increase interest, have a dance competition: whoever dances the longest wins. Those who are unable to stand can march their feet and swing their arms. Those that need supervision can dance with a staff member.

Walking can be another entertaining group activity. Help residents to set daily walking or self-propelling goals and map out 10-min walks within your site. Staff can set a specific destination, such as going for a cup of coffee or to see a garden beyond a window. Another activity is playing musical chairs. Put on some oldies music and have the residents walk or self-propel around a circle of chairs and sit when the music stops.

For residents who enjoyed housekeeping and caring for their homes, cleaning their rooms is an option. Give these residents the supplies and help them to start dusting and sweeping, clearing the dining room tables, or setting tables for the next meal. Incorporating an "it is never too late to play" philosophy, add horseshoes, croquet, flyswatter badminton, shuffleboard, and beanbag tosses to daily group activities within institutional settings.

For success, potential barriers to engaging residents in exercise activities must be recognized and addressed. These include comorbid conditions, fear of injury on the part of the resident as well as the health care team, pain, lack of suitable space and equipment, and lack of staff, resident, and family knowledge about the benefits of exercise and exercise options. In addition, there may be cognitive and motivational challenges (see Table 8.5).

Table 8.5 Overcoming barriers to engaging residents in exercise

Barrier	Intervention
Comorbidities	Optimize status of underlying conditions such as congestive heart failure, osteoarthritis, urinary incontinence
Fear of injury	Discuss fear and the ways to that resident injury will be prevented
Pain	Treat pain with nonpharmacological interventions or medications as needed [16]
Exercise equipment and opportunities	Create clear open pathways for walking and fun destination areas; consider purchasing resources via NASCO.com or other suppliers
Knowledge and beliefs of residents, families and staff	Repeated education and verbal encouragement for the residents; sharing information for families and staff via lay written materials and scholarly findings as relevant; and community newsletters for dissemination

Cognitive and Behavioral Problems

As many as 90% of older adults in long-term care facilities have some cognitive impairment with associated symptoms of aphasia, motor apraxia, perceptual impairments, and apathy. These conditions provide additional challenges to engaging residents in exercise or other types of physical activity. Furthermore, some individuals may have behavioral symptoms such as verbal or physical aggression, or resistance to care. Challenged by agitated or uncooperative behaviors of cognitively impaired residents, caregivers may focus on maintaining behavioral stability rather than engaging them in even basic functional tasks. This approach reinforces sedentary activity and a "just get it done" approach to personal care, in which the caregiver completes the functional task rather than supporting the resident to do so. Motivational "tricks of the trade" for caregivers are available on the Function Focused Care webpage (www.functionfocusedcare.org). This webpage houses six, 3-min video coaching sessions that demonstrate how to engage residents in exercise and functional activities in challenging situations. Written resources and ideas for exercise activities appropriate for institutionalized older adults are also available at this site. Additional examples include encouraging residents to walk to the hair salon; putting out small weights, foam balls, or elastic exercise bands in the dining room to spark residents or staff interest in spontaneous exercise; and developing a "function over fashion!" philosophy for your environments, by placing an exercycle, safe for older adults, in the dining area.

Motivation to Exercise

Along with cognitive and behavioral challenges, underlying motivation of the individual to exercise needs to be considered [17]. Figure 8.1 provides an overview of the many factors that can positively influence motivation to engage in exercise. Helping

Fig. 8.1 Factors that influence motivation to exercise in older adults

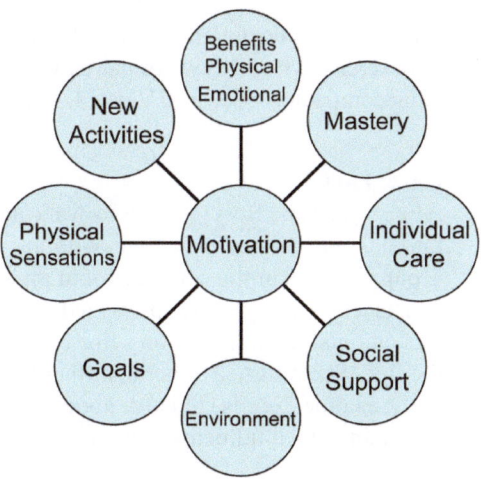

older adults as well as their caregivers to believe in the benefits of exercise is an important first step. Encouraging activities in which the individual will be successful and that will not cause discomfort or injury is important. Physical discomfort associated with exercise should be eliminated through modifications of activities and pretreatments (e.g., heat, acetaminophen, stretching). For example, stretching exercises will decrease the discomfort associated with disuse and long periods of sitting. Examples of activities may be viewed in videos provided in the Resource section.

Social supports and encouragement provided by others are important sources of motivation for older institutionalized adults. This encouragement should come from health care team members, families, and others who interact with the resident. Ongoing verbal encouragement to exercise, walk, go to an exercise class, or simply perform transfers is important. Even when residents refuse, often related to lack of self-efficacy, encouragement to engage in exercise should continue. Team members should not accept a final answer, but should continue to encourage participation in physical activities. Ongoing verbal encouragement can improve self-efficacy and underscore the importance of exercise, an activity as critical as taking one's medications, which receives substantial, repeated emphasis in institutional settings. Appropriate communication techniques and ensuring that the individual can hear and understand what is being said are also important [18].

While eliminating unpleasant sensations associated with exercise is essential, it is equally important to ensure that exercise is a pleasant experience. New and varied types of activities can engage individuals in exercise. For example, a new dance program, an evening prom, and "a walk across America" are ways to stimulate interest and enjoyment. Introducing lively music to group sit-to-stand exercises before mealtimes can add pleasure to this task.

To motivate older adults to exercise, individualized goals that take into consideration underlying physical and cognitive capability, and resident preferences are needed. Getting to know the individual and what types of exercise or work she did when younger will provide useful information to support motivation. For example, an older, retired nurse may be willing to walk the ward with you to make rounds. A retired television repair man or mailman may find interest in delivering televisions or the mail for you. Many older adults enjoy interacting with animals; a small study of assisted living residents demonstrated both increased gait speed and adherence to continued exercise when they were paired with a dog, from a local shelter, vs. a human walking companion. (See also Video 4.4 in Chap. 4, Pet Therapy Exercise Class).

Case: Part 3
After 6 months, Beryl is able to walk more than 100 feet at a time, without fatigue, and get out of a chair without assistance. She particularly enjoyed group sessions in the exercise room on a stationary bicycle, set at the lowest resistance, where the group was led on a different "trip" each day, and group relaxation/stretching sessions. She remarked "I feel stronger than before I had the flu!" She returned to her apartment with personal assistance several hours daily, a home exercise plan for good and bad weather days, and a commitment to obtain annual influenza immunization.

Conclusion

The benefits of exercise for older institutionalized adults outweigh potential associated risks. For each individual, the amount and intensity of exercise will vary and can be easily determined. What is perceived as a moderate level of aerobic activity by an institutionalized older adult often will be very different than that perceived as moderate intensity for healthy older adults. Individualized assessments to evaluate the resident's physical and cognitive abilities are important first steps in developing a suitable exercise plan. In addition, motivational techniques must be considered to ensure that the individual will engage in activities.

Implementing an innovative approach that focuses on optimizing the function and physical activity of older institutionalized adults rather than task completion is challenging. This approach requires a team and significant institutional commitment. Without question, exercise is the best "medicine" for institutionalized older adults and thus requires equal attention. Establishing individualized exercise goals that can be incorporated into daily life will promote attainment of the highest level of health and function for older institutionalized adults.

References

1. Courel-Ibáñez J, et al. Impact of tailored multicomponent exercise for preventing weakness and falls on nursing home residents' functional capacity. J Am Med Dir Assoc. 2022;23(1):98–9.
2. Zou Z, et al. The effect of group-based Otago exercise program on fear of falling and physical function among older adults living in nursing homes: a pilot trial. Geriatr Nurs. 2022;43:288–99.
3. Shuo W, et al. How exercise protects against mild cognitive impairment in nursing home-dwelling older adults: a path analysis. J Nerv Ment Dis. 2021;209(9):674–80.
4. Exercise is Medicine. Stay active even when feeling frail. 2021. https://www.exerciseis-medicine.org/assets/page_documents/Rx%20for%20health%20-%20staying%20active%20even%20when%20feeling%20frail.pdf.
5. Birimoglu Okuyan C, Deveci E. The effectiveness of Tai Chi Chuan on fear of movement, prevention of falls, physical activity, and cognitive status in older adults with mild cognitive impairment: a randomized controlled trial. Perspect Psychiatr Care. 2021;57(3):1273–81.
6. Wang S, et al. Effects of Chinese square dancing on older adults with mild cognitive impairment. Geriatr Nurs. 2020;41(3):290–6.
7. Exercise is Medicine®. Being active when you have osteoarthritis. 2019. https://www.exerciseismedicine.org/assets/page_documents/EIM_Rx%20for%20Health_Osteoarthritis.pdf.
8. Gebhard D, Mir E. What moves people living with dementia? Exploring barriers and motivators for physical activity perceived by people living with dementia in care homes. Qual Health Res. 2021;31(7):1319–34.
9. Heesterbeek M, van der Zee E, van Heuvelen M. Feasibility of three novel forms of passive exercise in a multisensory environment in vulnerable institutionalized older adults with dementia. J Alzheimers Dis. 2019;70(3):681–90.
10. Carlson J, et al. Interactions between psychosocial and built environment factors in explaining older adults' physical activity. Prev Med. 2012;54(1):68–73.
11. Resnick B, Galik E, Boltz M. Function focused care approaches: literature review of progress and future possibilities. J Am Med Dir Assoc. 2013;14:5.
12. Resnick, B. Function focused care interventions. 2022. www.functionfocusedcare.org.

13. Resnick B, et al. Physical capability scale: psychometric testing. Clin Nurs Res. 2013;22(1):7–29.
14. Chen T, et al. Dose-response association between accelerometer-assessed physical activity and incidence of functional disability in older japanese adults: a 6-year prospective study. J Gerontol Ser A Biol Sci Med Sci. 2020;75(9):1763–70.
15. Lu Z, et al. The U-shaped relationship between levels of bouted activity and fall incidence in community-dwelling older adults: a prospective cohort study. J Gerontol Ser A Biol Sci Med Sci. 2020;75(10):e145–51.
16. Levenson S, Resnick B. The AMDA pain CPG: a different kind of trustworthy clinical guideline. J Am Med Dir Assoc. 2021;22(12):2405–6.
17. Resnick B. The wheel that moves. Rehabil Nurs. 1994;19:140.
18. Mamo S, et al. A mixed methods study of hearing loss, communication, and social engagement in a group care setting for older adults. Persp ASHA Special Interest Groups. 2022;7(2):592–609.

Online Videos and Resources

Centers for Disease Control. Physical activity in older adults. 2022. https://www.cdc.gov/physicalactivity/basics/older_adults/.

Exercise is Medicine. Stay active even when feeling frail. 2021. https://www.exerciseismedicine.org/assets/page_documents/Rx%20for%20health%20-%20staying%20active%20even%20when%20feeling%20frail.pdf.

Exercise is Medicine®. Being active when you have osteoarthritis. 2019. https://www.exerciseismedicine.org/assets/page_documents/EIM_Rx%20for%20Health_Osteoarthritis.pdf.

Function Focused Care. www.functionfocusedcare.org.

NASCO Senior exercise and fitness. https://www.enasco.com/c/Senior-Activities-Nasco/Senior-Exercise-Fitness.

National Center on Health, Physical Activity, and Disability. For individuals and caregivers. https://www.nchpad.org/Individuals~Caregivers#video-1.

National Institute of Aging, Exercise & Physical Activity. Your everyday guide from the national institute on aging. http://www.nia.nih.gov/health/publication/exercise-physical-activity/introduction.

Rate of Pereived Exertion, Borg Scale. https://www.acsm.org/docs/current-comments/perceivedexertion.pdf.

US Department of Health and Human Services. Physical Activity guidelines for Americans: 2nd Edition. 2018. https://health.gov/sites/default/files/2019-09/Physical_Activity_Guidelines_2nd_edition.pdf#page=67.

Chapter 9
Promoting Mobility in the Acute Care Setting

Lobna Ali and Cynthia J. Brown

Key Points
- Older adults are at high risk for deconditioning as a result of bed rest and low mobility during hospitalization
- Deconditioning results in loss of function and discharge to higher levels of care, such as a nursing home, even after an elective or short emergency hospital stay
- Older adults can participate in walking, resistance exercises, and early rehabilitation programs without increasing adverse events during acute hospitalization
- Geriatric acute hospital units using comprehensive geriatric assessment, multidisciplinary teams, and interventions targeted to preserving function and mobility have the strongest evidence for reducing decline
- System-wide interventions, such as changing the default activity order to "out of bed" are recommended by experts

Case
Betty is an 82-year-old woman hospitalized from home after a few days' illness with fever and cough. She is admitted to the medical ward and treated with IV fluids, antibiotics, acetaminophen, and oxygen by nasal cannula for pneumonia. After 24 h, she is able to sit up in bed, talk, and eat 25–50% of her meals. Without her oxygen, she maintains adequate saturation and her oxygen is discontinued. She has a 5 cm red area on her sacrum, new since admission, which the nurse rates as a stage 1 pressure ulcer. While she has orders for out of bed as tolerated, Betty spends most of her hospital stay lying in bed; she

L. Ali · C. J. Brown (✉)
Louisiana State University Health Sciences Center, New Orleans, LA, USA
e-mail: lali@lsuhsc.edu; cbro50@lsuhsc.edu

© The Author(s), under exclusive license to Springer Nature
Switzerland AG 2024
G. M. Sullivan, A. K. Pomidor (eds.), *Exercise for Aging Adults*,
https://doi.org/10.1007/978-3-031-52928-3_9

feels a little unsteady when up and there are few staff to help her walk. Betty's nurses are afraid she might fall.

Prior to admission Betty was living on her own, with help from her family for groceries and transportation. She did not engage in specific exercise but was able to walk 100 feet to get her mail every day without an assistive device or difficulty. The day prior to discharge, physical therapy is called to evaluate Betty for post-discharge plans. They determine that she is too weak for discharge to home and recommend post-acute care rehabilitation until she is able to be safe on her own at home.

Introduction

Since the time of Hippocrates, clinicians have observed that prolonged low mobility, defined as bed rest or bed to chair activity, results in loss of muscle strength and function. In the 1940s Dr. Tinsley Harrison wrote of the abuse of rest when used as a therapeutic measure and recognized that this rest had unintended negative consequences. In the 1960s, the National Aeronautics and Space Administration (NASA) used head down bed rest to simulate space flight and documented significant changes in the healthy astronauts tested, including muscle wasting, bone density loss, and plasma volume loss, to name a few. Unfortunately, more recent study has demonstrated that older adults are more likely to experience these losses compared to younger adults, even during short hospital stays. Many clinicians have trained in care systems in which it is assumed, without question, that most older adults admitted for elective or emergent reasons will require a subsequent rehabilitation or nursing home stay to regain their baseline function. Yet studies show that interventions can break this cycle of low mobility, loss of strength, loss of function, and discharge to higher care, higher cost settings.

Barriers to implementation of these interventions include: fear of harming the older adult, myths that exercise or mobility will interfere with healing, nursing and rehabilitation resources targeted to keeping the patient in bed or wheelchair, particularly as a fall prevention measure, and staff lacking training. All of these barriers are amenable to education. This chapter will discuss the consequences of low mobility and interventions that are effective for older hospitalized adults.

Prevalence and Consequences of Low Mobility in the Acute Hospital

In the USA, individuals 65 years and older are 16% of the US population and twice as likely to require hospitalization compared to middle-aged adults. Nearly 17% of the 54 million older US adults were hospitalized at least once during 2019, compared to only 8% in the 45–64 year age group [1]. These numbers become more pronounced with older cohorts. Discharges to post-acute care (PAC) such as home health, an inpatient rehabilitation facility, or long-term care increase with age, with those 65 years or older accounting for 70% of discharges to PAC. Many of these transitions are due to functional decline, which is seen in at least 30% of all older adults discharged from the hospital. This functional decline is usually attributed to the acute illness and patient comorbidities, however, low mobility, defined as bed rest or bed to chair activity during hospitalization, has been shown to have a role in this functional loss.

Low mobility during hospitalization adversely affects many organ systems (Table 9.1), with a net result of overall functional loss. For older adults, deconditioning and functional loss begin by day 2 of hospitalization; thus, prevention protocols must start at or soon after hospital admission [2, 3]. Studies reveal that declines from baseline function in mobility and self-care are common, which often results in the need for new nursing home placement [4]. Studies have shown that, on average, hospitalized patients spent most of their hospital stay lying in bed, even though many patients walked independently upon admission. In studies the amount of out-of-bed activity was minimal, a result that has been reproduced in several other countries [5]. Importantly, although bed rest is common, chart review finds no medical reason for the observed bed rest in a majority of instances [4].

For those with preexisting functional or cognitive impairments, hospitalization presents additional challenges to maintaining independence and returning home. Older adults using assistive devices such as canes or walkers are more likely to have functional decline during hospitalization than those who do not. In one qualitative

Table 9.1 Consequences of bed rest and low mobility

System	Complication
Function	Decline in functional status from baseline
Musculoskeletal	Bone loss
	Muscle loss
	Contractures
	Decreased balance
	Fatigue, sense of exhaustion
Skin	Pressure ulcer
Cardiovascular	Orthostatic hypotension
	Decrease in cardiac output
	Deep vein thrombosis
Respiratory	Atelectasis
	Aspiration pneumonia
	Pulmonary embolus
Gastrointestinal	Constipation
Genitourinary	Urinary incontinence

study of hospital barriers to mobility, lack of available ambulatory devices was cited by both patients and nurses [6].

Older adults with dementia are more likely to experience substantial loss in instrumental of activities of daily living (IADL) and activities of daily living (ADL) during hospitalization. Regaining lost abilities is related to the severity of cognitive impairment. In addition, dementia is a major independent risk factor for acquiring delirium, or acute confusional state, during hospital admission. Delirium presents a critical obstacle to treating the index illness as well as maintaining mobility and function [6].

Studies of hospitalized older adults find that those who lose IADL and ADL function during a short hospitalization may not recover lost function even after 3–6 months of rehabilitation [7]. For some, continued functional decline is likely due to underlying medical conditions. For others, recovery is dependent upon rehabilitation efforts, which vary greatly. For individuals who are unable to tolerate 3 hours daily of formal therapy, home or skilled nursing facility are the usual sites for post-hospital rehabilitation, rather than a rehabilitation hospital. In the home or skilled nursing facility, older adults usually participate in a single exercise session from a few times weekly to daily. Particularly in institutional settings, staff may perform IADLs and ADLs for the older adult, to save time and reduce fall risk, which perpetuates continued decline in function (see Chap. 8).

Barriers to Hospital Mobility

Numerous barriers to hospital mobility have been identified and successful mobility programs must address these issues. Broadly, these barriers can be broken down into four key categories: *patient-related, treatment-related, institution-related, and attitudinal factors* (see Fig. 9.1). While some of these factors are not modifiable, such as illness severity and comorbidities that may make mobility more difficult, many of these factors are modifiable. For example, having ambulatory devices available on the hospital ward or minimizing the use of urinary catheters may reduce these potential barriers to mobility. Another important barrier is a lack of clarity regarding ownership of mobility during hospitalization. A 2022 systematic review of 48 studies identified the main barriers at the intrapersonal level to be physical health status, having lines or drains, patients' fear, and healthcare team's safety concerns. At the interpersonal level, the patient-health care team relationship and healthcare team's unclear roles were key. At the institutional level, this review found that the main barriers to mobility were lack of space and resources, including time and equipment [8]. In many hospitals physical therapy (PT) is identified as responsible for mobility. Yet, PT staffing is often inadequate to provide the necessary assistance with ambulation for all hospitalized patients. In fact, simply walking patients does not require the skills of a PT and could be delegated to other healthcare team members, with appropriate training.

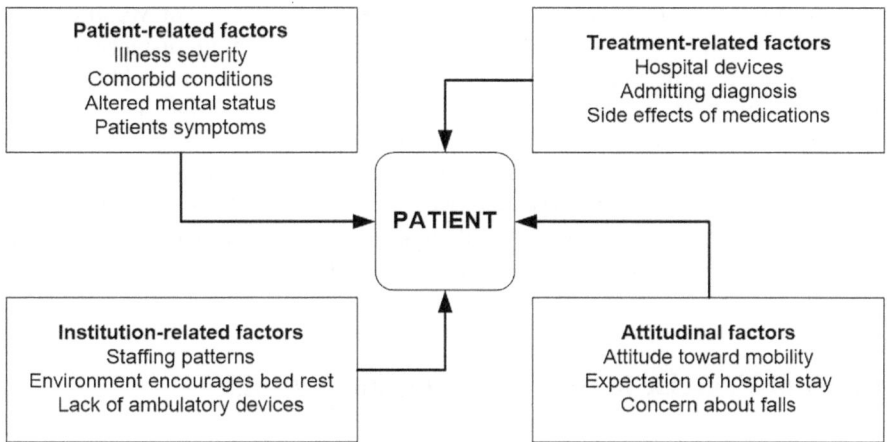

Fig. 9.1 Potential barriers to hospital mobility. Brown CJ, Williams BR, Woodby LL, Davis LL, Allman RM. Barriers to mobility during hospitalization from the perspectives of older patients and their nurses and physicians. J Hosp Med. 2007 Sep;2(5):305-13

Although low mobility in hospitalized older adults is common and associated with adverse health outcomes during and after hospitalization, it is often poorly recognized and inadequately addressed. Unfortunately, there is no consensus on mobility assessment in the inpatient setting and neither is there a mandate for implementing assessment tools. Hence, mobility is often missed as an important intervention in the healing and recovery for older hospitalized adults.

Assessing Function and Mobility in Hospitalized Older Adults

Fortunately, studies demonstrate that interventions can minimize hospital-associated functional decline [9]. A variety of approaches have shown benefit; most of these approaches start with an assessment of the older adult's preadmission function and risks for functional loss. Independent risk factors for hospital functional loss and nursing home placement include increasing age, low preadmission cognitive status, and low baseline IADL status; thus, these factors should be part of an intake assessment for older adults. In addition to the assessment of functional status, mobility also needs to be assessed.

Although several instruments are available to assess physical performance and mobility in older adults, none is considered ideal for all individuals or settings. Some mobility assessment tools that can be used in the hospital include the Banner Mobility Assessment Tool, which is completed by nursing and has four levels. Patients are asked to sit up and shake hands (level 1), Stretch and point (level 2), Stand (level 3), and Walk (level 4). Initial validity evidence showed a kappa statistic of 0.75 between the expert PT and the bedside nurse, which indicates adequate agreement [10]. Another tool is the Johns Hopkins Highest Level of Mobility scale. This tool is completed by nursing and documents the maximum distance a patient walks during a shift, and ranges from bed rest to 250 feet or more [11]. The de Morton Mobility Index (DEMMI) is a 15-item tool that examines bed and chair mobility, walking, and static and dynamic balance [12]. Scores range from 0 to 100 with higher scores indicating better mobility. The Hierarchical Assessment of Balance and Mobility (HABAM) scale rates balance (6 possible levels), transfers (8 levels), and mobility (14 levels). With this additional specificity, the HABAM instrument requires more time and training to use [13].

Safety of Exercise in the Acute Hospital Setting

To date studies, including pooled data in meta-analyses, have shown no increase in adverse effects, such as falls, injuries, or infections, in older adults engaged in hospital exercise programs [9, 14, 15]. No increase in adverse consequences is seen even with high-intensity resistance exercises performed in bed when compared with passive range of motion [16]. In fact, some programs show decreased hospital length of stay and decreased fall risk in the active intervention groups.

Studies have typically excluded older adults with unstable medical conditions as well as those in the intensive care unit (ICU) or receiving palliative care. Some programs exclude older adults who were not ambulatory prior to admission or who have been admitted from a nursing home. Other individuals who need additional review prior to entering a standard hospital mobility program are listed in Table 9.2.

Physical impairment, whether due to deconditioning or to acquiring the motor neuropathy syndrome known as *ICU-acquired weakness*, is common in adults who survive an ICU stay. Although few in number, randomized controlled studies of rehabilitation in the ICU setting demonstrate the feasibility and safety of physical therapy to improve immediate and long-term function [17]. In this setting, range of motion and bed mobility exercises are often initiated first. For selected patients, sitting exercise, transfers from bed to chair, resistance exercises, and ambulation are employed. Programs have successfully integrated reduced use of heavy sedation with physical and occupational therapy that starts within 72 h after intubation. Study results suggest benefits such as shorter ICU stays, earlier return to walking status, and greater likelihood of regaining baseline function.

Table 9.2 Older adults to exclude from standard approaches	
	Head trauma
	Spinal trauma
	Significant lower extremity trauma
	Hypotension
	Symptomatic tachyarrhythmias
	Active bleeding
	Unstable respiratory system

Promoting Mobility and Function with Geriatric Units and Teams

Traditionally, hospitals have focused on treating the acute illness or surgical procedure rather than considering the hazards of hospitalization for older adults. Thus, clinicians and staff focus on the principle reason for hospitalization—the pneumonia, fracture, myocardial infarction, or cholecystectomy—rather than overall function and independence, which primarily determines quality of life for older adults. Hospital administrators place considerable attention on the most efficient, rapid method to deliver care. Protocols may emphasize prevention of injuries, such as falls, rather than avoiding discharge to higher levels of care. The easiest way to avoid a fall or injury is to not permit mobility; thus many hospital policies actually promote muscle loss, decreased mobility, and loss of function.

Hospital geriatric teams and geriatric geographic units that employ geriatric assessment and individualized patient treatment plans have been extensively studied since the 1980s. Many studies have used rigorous study designs, with more than 22 randomized controlled trials, but have variable target patient groups, assessment instruments, interventions, and outcomes. Despite this heterogeneity, several meta-analyses have found that hospital-based geriatric units and teams are associated with improved function, mortality rates, and likelihood of returning home, and reduced likelihood of living in an institution [9, 15]. The number of older patients needed to treat (NNT) for the outcomes of survival and returning home ranges from 17 (home at 6 months after hospitalization) to 33 (home at 12 months after hospitalization), in comparison with usual medical care [9]. Benefits in reduced hospital costs are also seen; studies have not analyzed savings from fewer nursing home stays, which would further decrease costs.

In subgroup analyses comparing teams and geographic units, Ellis and colleagues found that specialized geriatric units were more effective than mobile geriatric teams, which have variable outcomes [9]. Only 13 (follow-up at 6 months) or 20 (12 months) older adults need to be treated in a geographic geriatric unit to prevent one person from dying or living in an institution [9]. Also, benefits are seen whether admission to the geriatric unit is based solely on age, such as 75 years and older; particular conditions, such as delirium or falls; or perceived needs, such as functional impairment or risk for institutionalization. Thus, comprehensive assessment delivered through a dedicated multidisciplinary team working in a geographically distinct unit improves an older adult's chance to survive hospitalization and return home.

One example of a specialized geriatrics unit is the *Acute Care of the Elderly* or ACE unit. These programs use geriatric assessment and multidisciplinary teams to deliver acute medical care while targeting interventions to maintain function. ACE units encourage patients to participate in ADLs and promote daily exercise, such as walking in hallways. Multidisciplinary teams conduct daily rounds that focus on function as well as medical concerns. Also, the environment of an ACE unit is designed to enhance mobility: handrails in unobstructed hallways, elevated toilets for easier transfer, and exercise space integrated into the unit.

Additional Hospital-Based Strategies

Age Friendly Health Care

The *age friendly health system* initiative seeks to ensure reliable application of four essentials of geriatric care at the health system level, not just within the hospital. The goal of the initiative is to enhance the care experience and improve satisfaction with care for older adults, reduce health-care related harm, reduce costs, and optimize value. These four evidence-based essentials, known as the "4Ms," provide the framework and include knowing and acting on what Matters to the older person, as well as a focus on Medications, Mentation, and Mobility. Specific to mobility, health systems are encouraged to screen for mobility across settings and to have plans in place to address low mobility if it is observed. As of May 2022, there are over 2800 recognized age friendly health system participants, however, studies demonstrating the effectiveness are currently lacking.

NICHE

Started in 1990, *Nurses Improving Care of Healthsystem Elders* (NICHE) is a national program to promote high-quality, evidence-based care of older adults. The project has developed and disseminated assessment tools, best practices, and educational materials for nurses. The most common NICHE strategy for improving the care of hospitalized older adults is the resource nurse model. In this strategy, assigned unit-based nurses acquire expertise in geriatrics best practices and disseminate information and skills to other nurses on the unit. Although this practical model makes sense, it is a more dilute intervention than the mobile geriatrics team and geographic geriatrics unit, and studies to date have not demonstrated consistent functional benefits.

Hospital Environments

Typically, hospital hallways have not been designed for patient ambulation but rather to move beds, equipment, and people as efficiently as possible. Similarly, rooms have not been arranged to facilitate walking to the bathroom or to a chair. IV poles, urinary catheters, and other devices tether patients in place. Bedrails, bed heights left elevated, and a multitude of equipment clutter the average room and environs. Areas suitable for safe walking can be created by adding nonglare lighting, railings, markers for distances walked, and periodic seating for rest stops. In addition, appropriate assistive devices, such as adjustable canes or walkers, can be available on units and patients trained in their use early in the hospital stay, not just on the day of discharge. Patients also need gowns that do not gap open, such as opposing johnny gowns, and nonslip footwear to facilitate mobility. Reduction of the use of urinary catheters and intravenous lines also make ambulation easier for the older adult.

Standardized Protocols or Order Sets

Orthopedics research has found that early mobilization programs—out of bed or walking on day of surgery—significantly reduces length of stay and improves joint function after hip or knee surgery, without increasing adverse outcomes and with retained patient satisfaction. Borrowing in part from these studies, hospitals have initiated walking programs for older adults.

Walking for Wellness [18] and *Project Move* [19] are examples of hospital-based programs that provide an overall framework for all older patients. These programs automatically provide a shared initial assessment, patient education, and mobility plans used across a hospital. Some of these programs have demonstrated reduced complications from low mobility as well as sustainability as a system-wide intervention. Trained escorts, family members, nurses, and physical therapists are used in these programs. Clarity, ease of operation, and consistency of implementation are essential elements of hospital-wide projects.

Another hospital-wide strategy is to eliminate "bed rest" as a default admission order. When bed rest is ordered as an add-on order, an explanation must be given by the ordering clinician. Analogous to restraint orders, bed rest orders can be allowed for only a short duration before expiration, such as 24 h, and must be reordered to be continued. This strategy has also been used in some ICU settings, in which the computerized order entry system no longer lists bed rest as the default activity level but does list physical and occupational therapist consultation, in automatically generated admission orders.

Ongoing hospital-wide education regarding the importance of patients continuing to perform self-care activities, sitting out of bed, and early mobilization is also recommended by experts. See Tables 9.3 and 9.4 for descriptions of hospital-based exercise interventions and approaches.

Over the past several years, significant interest has been paid toward making mobility an indicator of quality care. While somewhat more difficult to measure than number of falls or falls with injury, the outcomes associated with mobility or lack thereof are striking. The American Geriatrics Society published a white paper identifying the need for mobility during hospitalization to be better assessed and outlining a number of recommendations for health systems and the Center for Medicare and Medicaid Services (CMS) [20] (see Table 9.5). The CMS Innovation project targeted hospital mobility in 300+ hospitals with a focus on educating healthcare providers and providing a toolkit to encourage assessment of mobility as well as targeted interventions. Finally, many organizations are advocating for a change in focus from fall prevention to safe mobility.

Table 9.3 Hospital interventions for older adults

Type	Interventions	Outcomes
Geographic geriatrics unit	Comprehensive geriatric assessment Dedicated geriatrics team Daily discussion of function Protocols for geriatric conditions Enhanced environments	Reduced discharge to higher levels of care
		Better function
		Reduced mortality
		Better cognitive status at discharge
		Reduced costs, length of stay
Mobile geriatrics team	Comprehensive geriatric assessment	Variable
	Geriatrics consult team	
	Recommendations focused on geriatric conditions and function	
Unit-based nurse resource	Nurse with enhanced knowledge and experience in geriatrics best practices	Few studies: little differences
	Educational materials such as assessments targeting common geriatrics conditions	
Early physical rehabilitation	Multidisciplinary programs with exercise component or usual care with exercise program Exercise 5 times/week, up to 2 times daily, with focus on strength, mobility, and balance	Variable: most studies show improved physical function tests and some show reduced discharge to nursing home
		No increase in injuries, falls, or adverse events
		Most patients adhere to program
Walking programs	*Walking for Wellness* [18]: trained escorts (from transportation staff) supervise patients' daily walking in hallways 2–3 times/day, patient brochures and short video, family education, walking aids such as canes and walkers, walking goals and walking record	High acceptance by patients
		High patient and family satisfaction
		Average 2 walks/day
	Project Move [19]: enhanced clarity of nurse and physical therapist roles, staff education, patient function included in nurse assessments and change-of-shift reports, stickers for patients "Ask Me if I Walked Today" and educational brochures for families, default order changed to "out of bed with progressive activity as tolerated," specific patient activity schedule	Physical therapy (PT) and occupational therapy (OT) perceived improved appropriateness of consults
		No increase in total PT or OT consults
		Decrease in pneumonia and pulmonary complications vs. prior 4 years
		Patients and families found program acceptable

Table 9.4 Components of hospital-wide approaches

Patient baseline and current function and mobility assessed on admission and daily
Functional information shared among clinical staff, including nurses, physical therapists, and physicians, such as during handovers, huddles, and interdisciplinary discharge rounds
Set mobility goals daily with patient/family and document progress toward goal in a visible place (i.e., whiteboard)
Eliminate bed rest orders as the default order; the default order is out of bed daily and walk each shift
Involve patients and family members in exercise activities
Assistive mobility devices available on admission
Ongoing monitoring of the environment's role in encouraging exercise activities, such as walking
Ongoing tracking and reporting of statistics measuring patients requiring higher level of care environments at discharge, as compared with before admission
Ongoing clinical staff education about the hazards of immobility

Table 9.5 AGS quality and performance measurement committee recommendations to integrate mobility programs into hospital care for older adults

Recommendation	Suggest	Responsible organizers/ stakeholders	Performance incentives/compliance motivation
1	Promote mobility assessment in acute care	CMS	Provide incentives for the use of standard, validated mobility assessments that are harmonized with other mandated assessments to minimize the work burden placed on care providers
2	Advocate for more research funding	Federal Agencies, e.g., AHRQ, NIH-NIA	Prioritize translational research in mobility assessment Quality measurement Implementation of mobility intervention programs
3	Develop consensus on standard methods to assess mobility	CMS Other stakeholders	Promote development of consensus on an assessment that is – Valid – Appropriate for acute care settings – Clinically meaningful to clinicians and patients
4	Minimize the burden of mobility measurement	Healthcare institution-hospital	Focus on optimizing workflow and documentation, and minimizing redundancy by – Specifying roles of healthcare professionals, such as nurses and physical therapists – Use of existing clinical data in the health record – Use of innovative technological solutions

(continued)

Table 9.5 (continued)

Recommendation	Suggest	Responsible organizers/ stakeholders	Performance incentives/compliance motivation
5	Evaluate the feasibility of a mobility quality measure	CMS	Develop a mobility quality measure to encourage hospitals, staff, and clinicians to intervene, to prevent loss of mobility in hospitalized older adults
6	Reframe the current regulatory focus on falls in acute care to a focus on safe mobility	Hospital system	With little evidence of the effectiveness of strategies to prevent falls in acute care, reconsider use falls or falls with injury as quality indicators, in the absence of a balancing measure for mobility
7	Develop resources for acute care clinicians	AGS Strategic partners	Create tools, processes, strategies to assist clinicians and hospitals with rapid, efficient, sustainable implementation of evidence-based practices for mobility assessment and intervention

AGS American Geriatrics Society, *CMS* Centers of Medicare and Medicaid Services, *AHRQ* Agency for Healthcare Research and Quality, *NIH-NIA* National Institutes of Health – National Institute of Aging
Adopted from: Wald, H. L., Ramaswamy, R., Perskin, M. H., Roberts, L., Bogaisky, M., Suen, W., ... & Quality and Performance Measurement Committee of the American Geriatrics Society. (2019). The case for mobility assessment in hospitalized older adults: American Geriatrics Society white paper executive summary. *Journal of the American Geriatrics Society, 67*(1), 11-16 [20]

Conclusion

Older adults are at particularly high risk for consequences of immobility due to hospitalization. Feared yet common outcomes are loss of physical function, mobility, and discharge to a higher level of care rather than home. Older age and prior cognitive and IADL impairments are associated with greater risk for these outcomes. Traditionally, hospitals have focused on the acute illness more than the hazards of hospitalization experienced by older patients. Yet research in the hospital setting reveals opportunities to prevent deconditioning and loss of function in older adults.

The most valuable intervention appears to be the geographic, multidisciplinary geriatrics unit, which may also reduce hospital costs. However, simple walking programs with trained escorts or family members can increase amount of time walking and out of bed greatly, and are safe and acceptable to patients and families. Similarly, order sets that default to "out-of-bed" activity status will greatly reduce the time in bed. Many clinicians accept the cycle of hospitalization, muscle weakness, functional loss, nursing home stay, and rehospitalization as inevitable. Indeed, this may be true for older adults at highest risks of decline, but greater adoption of hospital "best practices," such as ACE units. will break this cycle for many hospitalized older adults.

References

1. 2020 profile of older Americans. 2021. https://acl.gov/sites/default/files/aging%20 and%20Disability%20In%20America/2020Profileolderamericans.final_pdf. Accessed 16 December 2022.
2. Hirsch CH, Sommers L, Olsen A, et al. The natural history of functional morbidity in hospitalized older adults. J Am Geriatr Soc. 1990;38:1296–303.
3. Mudge AM, O'Rourke P, Denaro CP. Timing and risk factors for functional changes associated with medical hospitalization in older patients. J Gerontol A Biol Sci Med Sci. 2010;65:866–72.
4. Brown CJ, Friedkin RJ, Inouye SK. Prevalence and outcomes of low mobility in hospitalized older patients. J Am Geriatr Soc. 2004;52(8):1263–70.
5. Brown CJ, Redden DT, Flood KL, Allman RM. The underrecognized epidemic of low mobility during hospitalization of older adults. J Am Geriatr Soc. 2009;57(9):1660–5.
6. Brown CJ, Williams BR, Woodby LL, Davis LL, Allman RM. Barriers to mobility during hospitalization from the perspectives of older patients and their nurses and physicians. J Hosp Med. 2007;2(5):305–13.
7. Li X, Zheng T, Guan Y, Li H, Zhu K, Shen L, Yin Z. ADL recovery trajectory after discharge and its predictors among baseline-independent older inpatients. BMC Geriatr. 2020;20(1):86.
8. Dijkstra F, van der Sluis G, Jager-Wittenaar H, Hempenius L, Hobbelen JSM, Finnema E. Facilitators and barriers to enhancing physical activity in older patients during acute hospital stay: a systematic review. Int J Behav Nutr Phys Act. 2022;19(1):99.
9. Ellis G, Whitehead MA, Robinson D, et al. Comprehensive geriatric assessment for older adults admitted to hospital: meta-analysis of randomised controlled trials. BMJ. 2011;343:d6553.
10. Boynton T, Kelly L, Perez A, et al. Banner mobility assessment tool for nurses: instrument validation. Am J Safe Patient Handl Mov. 2014;4:86–92.
11. Johns Hopkins Medicine. OACIS: Resources–instruments and methods; 2018. Available at https://www.hopkinsmedicine.org/pulmonary/research/outcomes_after_critical_illness_surgery/oacis_instruments.html. Accessed 16 December 2022.
12. de Morton NA, Davidson M, Keating JL. Validity, responsiveness and theminimal clinically important difference for the de Morton Mobility Index(DEMMI) in an older acute medical population. BMC Geriatr. 2010;10:72.
13. Rockwood K, Rockwood MRH, Andrew MK, et al. Reliability of the hierarchical assessment of balance and mobility in frail older adults. J Am Geriatr Soc. 2008;56(7):1213–7.
14. Kosse NM, Dutmer AL, Dasenbrock L, Bauer JM, Lamoth CJ. Effectiveness and feasibility of early physical rehabilitation programs for geriatric hospitalized patients: a systematic review. BMC Geriatr. 2013;13:107.
15. Hartley P, Keating JL, Jeffs KJ, Raymond MJM, Smith TO. Exercise for acutely hospitalised older medical patients. Cochrane Database Syst Rev. 2022;11:CD005955. https://doi.org/10.1002/14651858.CD005955.pub3. Accessed 15 December 2022.
16. Mallery LH, MacDonald EA, Hubley-Kozey CL, Earl ME, Rockwood K, MacKnight C. The feasibility of performing resistance exercise with acutely ill hospitalized older adults. BMC Geriatr. 2003;3:3.
17. Lang JK, Paykel MS, Haines KJ, Hodgson CL. Clinical practice guidelines for early mobilization in the ICU: a systematic review. Crit Care Med. 2020;48(11):e1121–8.
18. Tucker D, Molsberger SC, Clark A. Walking for wellness: a collaborative program to maintain mobility in hospitalized older adults. Geriatr Nurs. 2004;25(4):242–5.

19. Markey DW, Brown RJ. An interdisciplinary approach to addressing patient activity and mobility in the medical-surgical patient. J Nurs Care Qual. 2002;16(4):1–12.
20. Wald HL, Ramaswamy R, Perskin MH, Roberts L, Bogaisky M, Suen W, Quality and Performance Measurement Committee of the American Geriatrics Society. The case for mobility assessment in hospitalized older adults: American Geriatrics Society white paper executive summary. J Am Geriatr Soc. 2019;67(1):11–6.

Resources

Age Friendly Healthsystem to reliably provide a set of four evidence-based elements of high-quality care, known as the "4Ms," to all older adults in your system: what matters, medication, mentation, and mobility. https://www.ihi.org/Engage/Initiatives/Age-Friendly-Health-Systems/Pages/default.aspx. Accessed 16 December 2022.

Ogrinc GS, Headrick LA, Barton AJ, Dolansky MA, Madigosky WS, Miltner RS, Hall AG. Fundamentals of health care improvement: a guide to improving your patients' care. 4th ed. Oakbrook Terrace: Joint Commission Resources and Institute for Healthcare Improvement; 2022. https://www.ihi.org/resources/Pages/Publications/fundamentals-of-health-care-improvement-a-guide-to-improving-your-patients-care.aspx. Accessed 16 December 2022.

Hospital Elder Life Program (HELP) program to reduce delirium in hospitalized older adults, which prevents functional loss. https://help.agscocare.org/. Accessed 16 December 2022.

Nurses Improving Care for Healthsystem Elders (NICHE) for reducing hospital functional decline. https://nicheprogram.org/. Accessed 16 December 2022.

Chapter 10
Community-Based Exercise Programs for Older Adults

Jennifer S. Brach and Gardenia A. Juarez

Key Points
- Community-based programs are designed to reach people outside the traditional healthcare setting, in "real world" settings
- Community-based programs have been shown to increase the time and the frequency of physical activity in older adults
- Community partnerships are critical to the sustainability of a community-based program
- Evidence-based programs increase the likelihood of a positive outcome, lead to efficient use of resources, and make it easier to justify funding
- The RE-AIM framework is a comprehensive framework for program planning and evaluation

Case

Mary is 82 years old, recently fell, and fractured her wrist. She is receiving physical therapy to restore her range of motion, strength, and function after the fracture. She reports being fearful of falling and is worried she may fall again and next time break her hip. She asks her physical therapist for recommendations.

Mary's physical therapist evaluates her mobility and determines she could benefit from a program to address her fear of falling and reduce her fall risk. She suggests that Mary continue exercising once her physical therapy sessions end, and identifies two programs offered at her local community center to address her needs: *A Matter of Balance* and *Enhance Fitness*.

J. S. Brach (✉) · G. A. Juarez
University of Pittsburgh, Pittsburgh, PA, USA
e-mail: jbrach@pitt.edu; gaj34@pitt.edu

© The Author(s), under exclusive license to Springer Nature Switzerland AG 2024
G. M. Sullivan, A. K. Pomidor (eds.), *Exercise for Aging Adults*,
https://doi.org/10.1007/978-3-031-52928-3_10

Mary decides to start with A Matter of Balance to learn practical, coping strategies to reduce fear of falling and for fall prevention. Once she completes the Matter of Balance program she will enroll in the ongoing Enhance Fitness program to maintain and improve her flexibility, endurance, strength, and balance. Mary is motivated to continue in the program as she sees improvement and enjoys socializing with the group after sessions.

Introduction

In older adults, physical activity and exercise can prevent mobility disability, hospitalization, and institutionalization as well as improve physical and mental health. Despite these benefits, the older adult age group engages in the least amount of moderate-to-vigorous physical activity and the most time in sedentary behavior, compared to other age groups. One attractive way to promote exercise is through community-based programs. Community-based programs take what we know from research and make that knowledge usable by public health and aging services teams. The idea is to take a research model which has been shown to work in the laboratory and to adapt it for use in the "real world."

Community-based programs are designed to reach people outside the traditional healthcare setting. These settings may include schools, worksites, community centers, congregate living areas, and churches. These nontraditional settings can encourage informal information sharing within communities through peer social interactions and social support. This is represented in the case as Mary is transitioning from receiving care in a traditional healthcare setting (physical therapy) to programs in her community. Mary selected programs in her community that address her fear of falling and ongoing exercise needs.

An excellent example of a community-based program occurring outside the traditional healthcare setting is the *Sisters in Motion* program [1]. The goal of this faith-based intervention is to increase walking among older, sedentary African American women. The multi-component program, which includes scripture readings, prayer, goal-setting, a community resource guide, and walking competitions, is delivered through churches in the Los Angeles area. The program has been successful in producing an increase in walking and a decrease in systolic blood pressure at 6 months. The use of settings outside the traditional healthcare setting is critical for serving hard to reach populations. The *Sisters in Motion* program is a great option for older African Americans who may not be exposed to community centers that offer physical activity programs but are likely to attend church regularly.

Community-based exercise programs for older adults have several benefits. Group-based community exercise programs for older adults can increase time spent exercising, the frequency of exercise, and aerobic capacity. However, less is known about the health cost implications of these programs. Ackermann et al. conducted a matched cohort study to determine if healthcare costs for Medicare-eligible adults who chose to participate in a community-based exercise program were different from individuals who did not participate in the community-based programs [2]. They found the average increase in annual total healthcare costs was less in those who participated in the community-based exercise program; if these findings are confirmed in other studies, group-based exercise programs could play a role in reducing overall health care costs.

Translation of Research into Evidence-Based Community Programs

Translating successful research findings into practice is critical if others outside research programs are to benefit. The goal is to bridge the gap between academic clinical research on exercise and the community. In the past decade, the aging network has increasingly implemented evidence-based health promotion programs. In fact, the Federal FY-2012 Congressional appropriations law includes an evidence-based requirement for all health promotion programs funded by Older Americans Act (OAA) Title IIID funds. In response to this requirement, the Administration on Aging (AOA) developed an evidence-based definition to assist leaders in identifying evidence-based programs. Programs are considered evidence-based if they meet the criteria in Box 10.1 As of 1 October 2016, Title IIID funds can only be used for health promotion programs that meet this definition of evidence-based programs.

Box 10.1 Definition of an Evidence-Based Health Promotion Community Program

Demonstrated through evaluation to be effective for improving the health and well-being or reducing disease, disability and/or injury among older adults; *and*

Proven effective with older adult population, using experimental or quasi-experimental designs; *and*

Research results published in a peer-reviewed journal; *and*

Fully translated in one or more community site(s); *and*

Includes developed dissemination products that are available to the public.

Why this major switch to evidence-based programs? There are several perceived advantages of evidence-based programs. These programs increase the likelihood of a positive outcome, are a more efficient use of resources, and make funding more easily justified. The push for evidence-based programming is coming from funders, agency leaders, and older adults themselves. Funders are increasingly demanding that programming be based on research evidence, agency leaders want to appropriate limited resources for proven programs, and older adults are looking for programs that are known to work.

The National Council on Aging, Center for Healthy Aging has developed a series of tools and checklist to assist individuals in the translation process from research evidence to practical, effective community-based programs. The National Council on Aging, Center for Healthy Aging has described the basic components of evidence-based health promotion planning (see Box 10.2).

Box 10.2 Basic Planning Components of Evidence-Based Health Promotion Planning

Identification of an important health issue and population at risk.
Identification of effective interventions.
Establishing broad-based partnerships within the community.
Selecting an intervention from the identified effective interventions.
Translating the intervention into a program.
Implementing the translated program.
Evaluating the program.
Sustaining the program.
From the National Council on Aging, Center for Healthy Aging [3].

The first component, *identification of an important health issue*, involves reviewing the literature, examining epidemiologic data, and talking to individuals within the community to identify a key health condition or risk factor that is pertinent for older adults in this community. Examples of health conditions or risk factors pertinent to older adults are injurious falls, pre-diabetes or diabetes mellitus, and hypertension.

Once a condition or risk factor is identified, the next step is to *identify effective interventions*. This is done by systematically searching and reviewing the research relevant to the health condition or risk factor. At this point it is helpful to identify several potential programs that address the health condition or risk factor. If not already involved in the process, this is an optimal time to establish partnerships within the community. Community partners are critical to determine the priorities of the population. Partners can also help to identify other relevant community stakeholders who should have early input into the process.

The next step is to *select* a proven, evidence-based intervention from the previously identified interventions. The selected intervention should be appropriate for the target population, suitable for adoption by the community health team, and feasible given the available resources. When selecting the program consider these needs: time to run the program, materials and equipment, available personnel, training, and program and training costs. These factors will influence selection of an intervention.

Once the intervention is identified and approved by all stakeholders it needs to be *translated* into a program suitable for implementation in the community, while maintaining fidelity to the key components of the intervention. It is important to ensure the translation of the evidence-based intervention into a community program remains a faithful and accurate representation of the original program.

After the intervention has been translated into operational steps, the program should be *piloted* in the community. To obtain an accurate trial run of the program, it is essential to test the new program in a group of older adults who are similar to the target population and may benefit from the intervention. For example, if the target population is sedentary older adults, it is important to implement the program in a group of sedentary older adults and not in a group of senior athletes. After piloting, some modifications to the original plan may be required. However, it is imperative to maintain the key or core concepts of the program when adapting to the target population and available community resources.

Prior to fully implementing the program, it is critical to have a plan in place for *evaluation*. This may require designing new or adapting existing instruments, such as surveys, for data collection. With new programs one may want to obtain feedback from the participants midway through the program so that the information can be used to make ongoing program adjustments. At the completion of the program, evaluate process measures, such as drop-out rates and satisfaction of participants with the delivery of the program, and key outcomes. The outcomes assessed should match the target of the intervention (i.e., if the goal is to increase physical activity, then amount of physical activity should be measured at completion of the program). Information from this final evaluation can be used to inform the next cycle of program planning.

The final step in the process is to ensure *sustainability* of the program. Throughout the translation process one should collect information on the activities and resources needed to maintain a successful program. Issues to consider include staff, space, resources, and materials. Partnerships that have been developed throughout the process can be key in the maintenance and sustainability of programs. Ongoing evaluation and modifications are needed to ensure that the program continues to meet the interests and needs of the target population.

Community Program Planning Steps

There are four main steps involved in program planning or implementation of an evidence-based program in the community (see Box 10.3) [4]. The first step is selecting an evidence-based program that works for the target community, as described above. Resources such as the National Council on Aging's Center for Healthy Aging, Administration for Community Living Title III-D list of evidence-based programs, Centers for Disease Control, and Evidence-Based Leadership Council can be used to identify programs. When evaluating potential evidence-based community programs, consider these questions: (1) is the program based on best practices; (2) was the program tested with a rigorous research design; (3) is the program effective for the outcomes of interest; (4) are there protocols and manuals available so that the program can be easily replicated; (5) has the program been tested in multiple settings and populations; (6) has it been published in peer-reviewed literature; and (7) is it feasible to scale up to a larger population?

Box 10.3 Community Program Planning Steps
1. Selecting a program
2. Determining readiness
3. Using RE-AIM to plan
4. Working with partners

The next component of program planning is determining the readiness of your organization to implement the program. The National Council on Aging has an online *Innovation Readiness Assessment* link that can be used to determine if an organization is ready. Factors that contribute to the readiness of an organization to implement a program include willingness to stay true to the program (i.e., program fidelity), available funding for the program, access to personnel to run the program, access to the target population who need the program, and buy in from senior leadership and key partners that is reflected in both programmatic and financial support.

The next stage is planning the intervention. One framework used to plan new interventions, adapt existing interventions, and design evaluations to assess potential health impacts is RE-AIM (www.re-aim.org). RE-AIM is a comprehensive framework that was developed by Glasgow et al. [5]. The evolving framework focuses on five critical elements: **R**each, **E**ffectiveness, **A**doption, **I**mplementation, and **M**aintenance (RE-AIM). These five elements are defined:

Reach—the absolute number, proportion, and representativeness of the persons who participate in a given program.
Effectiveness—the impact of the program on important outcomes.
Adoption—the absolute number, proportion, and representativeness of settings that are willing to offer the program.
Implementation—the degree to which staff members follow the program as designed (consistency, fidelity).
Maintenance—the extent in which the program becomes part of the routine in the setting of interest and at the level of the individual.

The final step in implementing community programs is establishing partnerships within the community. Without the support of community partners, programs are unlikely to be successful. Partnerships are crucial at every stage of the process (planning, implementation, evaluation, and sustaining) and should be identified early and maintained throughout the process. Community partners can make or break a program and it is critical to identify key partners to ensure successful programming.

Examples of Evidence-Based Community Exercise Programs for Older Adults

Community groups offer various evidence-based exercise programs to older adults such as programs for health promotion, self-management of chronic diseases, and fall prevention [6]. There are many evidence-based community exercise programs for older adults; five examples are presented here. These have different goals: fall reduction; improved fitness; improved balance, strength and endurance; improved mobility and motor control of walking; and improved whole body functional performance. Information on additional programs can be found on the Centers for Disease Control and Prevention (CDC: www.cdc.gov) and the National Council on Aging (NCOA: www.ncoa.org) websites.

A Matter of Balance (MOB), www.mainehealth.org/mob

The MOB program was designed to reduce fall risk and fear of falling in older adults, 60+ years of age, who are ambulatory, able to problem solve, concerned about falling, and want to increase their flexibility, balance, and strength. The class is delivered by two coaches who are volunteer lay leaders trained to teach the program. The program consists of 8 weekly, 2 h sessions. or twice weekly, 1-h sessions for a total of 16 h of instruction. The program emphasizes practical coping strategies to reduce fear of falling and teaches fall prevention strategies. The instructional group activities include group discussions, problem-solving, videos, sharing practical solutions, and exercise training. Coaches are required to attend 8 h of initial training and 2.5 h of annual update training in order to lead the program. The MOB program is a national program with over 500 Master Trainer Sites located in 39 states and the District of Columbia.

Enhance Fitness, www.projectenhance.org/EnhanceFitness.aspx

The primary goal of the Enhance Fitness program is to improve the overall functional fitness and well-being of older adults. The program was designed for sedentary older adults wishing to improve their physical functioning. Enhance Fitness is currently offered in hundreds of locations in the USA. The program is an ongoing, 1 h, 3 times per week group physical activity program that focuses on stretching and flexibility, low impact aerobics, strength training, and balance. The classes are led by certified fitness instructors who have completed 1.5 day Enhance Fitness new instructor training.

The Otago Exercise Program, www.med.unc.edu/aging/cgec/exercise-program

The Otago Exercise Program was originally developed in New Zealand. The goal of the program is to increase strength, balance, and endurance in community-dwelling frail older adults who are 65 years of age and older. The program was designed to be delivered at home, independently or with assistance, or in outpatient settings including assisted living facilities and community-based organizations. The older adult is evaluated by a physical therapist. The physical therapist selects 17 different exercises specifically for the older adult to do over the 8-week program, 3-times a week, for 30 min. The exercises progress as the individual gets stronger. If the older adult is strong enough to walk, a walking program can be offered up to 30 min, 3-times a week.

On the Move (OTM), www.onthemove.pitt.edu

The OTM program was developed at the University of Pittsburgh. It is a group-based exercise program for older adults designed to improve mobility by targeting key principles of the biomechanics and motor control of walking. Classes are 50 min in duration and held twice a week, for 12 weeks. The program contains a warm-up, stepping patterns, walking patterns, strengthening exercises, and cool-down exercises. Walking and stepping patterns are goal-oriented and progress in difficulty to continually challenge participants. The program is led by certified OTM instructors who are health professionals (physical therapists, physical therapy assistants, occupational therapists, and certified occupational therapy assistant) or certified fitness instructors in licensed facilities.

Bingocize, www.wku.edu/bingocize/

The Bingocize program was developed at Western Kentucky University. The main goals of this program for older adults are to: improve whole body functional performance, including gait, balance, and range of motion; executive cognitive function; social engagement; and knowledge of fall risk reduction. The 10-week program is offered twice weekly for 1 hour and combines the game of bingo with exercise and fall prevention. Bingocize also offers an optional mobile app which includes fall prevention and other health education topics. The program is led by certified staff or volunteer leaders of the licensed facility.

Delivery of Evidence-Based Programs

During the COVID-19 pandemic, all systems were forced to pivot and offer services remotely. Some evidence-based program creators and instructors opted to offer their programs in a virtual format. The virtual delivery of programs was well received by participants. As restrictions have lifted, the virtual delivery of programs has continued. Virtual programs reach individuals who otherwise may not be able to engage in exercise programs because of issues with access to or availability of programs, transportation, health restrictions, or caregiving responsibilities. Some individuals prefer virtual delivery because the exercises can be done in the comfort of their own home: they have no travel worries, they can access programs in other communities, and costs are low.

There are many evidence-based programs that target different populations (e.g., more frail or more robust) and have different goals (e.g., fall prevention or general fitness). Programs should not be used in isolation but should complement one another as is seen in our case. Mary begins with A Matter of Balance (MOB). Through MOB Mary reduces her fear of falling and practices fall prevention strategies. Mary is now ready to participate in another program, Enhance Fitness, to maintain and improve her flexibility, endurance, strength, and balance. Mary selected Enhance Fitness as it was available in her community and had a virtual option. The virtual option was appealing for times when the weather is inclement or she is busy with caregiving responsibilities.

Evidence-based programs are not meant to replace formal or traditional healthcare but can be used to extend and complement care. As demonstrated in the case, Mary used a community-based program at the conclusion of her formal physical therapy. This was convenient as it was located close to home and affordable. Transitions can work in the opposite direction as well. Instructors of community-based programs can recognize participants who are declining over time and make recommendations for further evaluation by the participant's healthcare clinician.

Conclusions

Community-based programs, delivered outside the traditional healthcare setting in locations such as community centers, congregate living areas, and churches, can promote physical activity in older adults. Many factors such as the goals of the program, resources required to run the program, and efficacy of the intervention should be considered when selecting a program. Funders and agency leaders are increasingly demanding evidence-based programs because they increase the likelihood of a positive outcome, lead to efficient use of resources, support continuous quality improvement, and make it easier to justify funding. A variety of evidence-based programs have been implemented in community settings and can serve as models for interested communities and leaders.

References

1. Duru OK, Sarkisian CA, Leng M, Mangione CM. Sisters in motion: a randomized trial of a faith-based physical activity intervention. J Am Geriatr Soc. 2012;58:1863–9.
2. Ackerman RT, Cheadle A, Sandhu N, Madsen L, Wagner EH, LoGerfo JP. Community exercise program use and changes in healthcare costs for older adults. Am J Prev Med. 2003;25:232–7.
3. The National Council on Aging. NCOA.org. https://www.ncoa.org/professionals/health/center-for-healthy-aging/. Accessed 17 July 2023.
4. Belza B, PRC-HAN Physical Activity Conference Planning Workgroup. Moving ahead: strategies and tools to plan, conduct, and maintain effective community-based physical activity programs for older adults. Atlanta: Centers for Disease Control and Prevention; 2007.
5. Glasgow RE, Vogt TM, Boles SM. Evaluating the public health impact of health promotion interventions: the RE-AIM framework. Am J Public Health. 1999;89(9):1922–7.
6. Brach JS, Juarez G, Perera S, Cameron K, Vincenzo JL, Tripken J. Dissemination and implementation of evidence-based falls prevention programs: reach and effectiveness. J Gerontol Ser A Biol Sci Med Sci. 2022;77(1):164–71. https://doi.org/10.1093/gerona/glab197.

Chapter 11
Exercise Adaptations for Older Athletes

Gail M. Sullivan and Jacob Earp

Key Points
- In the absence of disease or injury, on average, older athletes exercising at high levels experience slow declines in performance to age 75 years, with greater declines thereafter
- Muscle mass, power, and cardiovascular performance decline with age and may be partially reversible
- Older adults require more recovery time after "hard" work outs
- Cross-training is useful for promoting recovery and may help maintain the motivation to exercise
- Warms-ups, cool-downs, and stretching are frequently recommended for older athletes

Case: Part 1

Ann has always exercised at a high level, with extended bicycle and cross-country ski trips and many other sports. Now 79 years old, she's had two knee replacements and notes major problems with her balance: she feels she may fall when skiing. Her 82-year-old husband Davis, a competitive swimmer all his life, swims for exercise. He currently competes with and coaches an older adult swim team. Several times he has noted lightheadedness, briefly, after he completed a fast race and while still in the pool. He feels quite stiff and achy the day after a race. They want to continue their activities as long as possible and would like some advice.

G. M. Sullivan (✉)
UConn Center on Aging, University of Connecticut School of Medicine,
Farmington, CT, USA
e-mail: gsullivan@uchc.edu

J. Earp
Department of Kinesiology, University of Connecticut, Storrs, CT, USA
e-mail: jacob.earp@uconn.edu

© The Author(s), under exclusive license to Springer Nature   155
Switzerland AG 2024
G. M. Sullivan, A. K. Pomidor (eds.), *Exercise for Aging Adults*,
https://doi.org/10.1007/978-3-031-52928-3_11

Introduction

As the population—in numbers and percentage—of older adults continues to grow world-wide, health professionals will increasingly interact with and counsel the sub-group known as *master athletes*. Elite late life athletes, particularly those doing endurance and mixed sports, live longer, which may relate to their exercise habits among many other factors [1]. This elite group has been highly studied to understand aging physiology and physical performance that exclude the effects of a sedentary lifestyle [2]. In the sports world, master or senior athlete usually refers to those aged 35 years and older [2, 3]. These individuals exercise at a greater frequency, 5–6 times weekly, and intensity than most persons their age. They continue to compete as well, locally, nationally, or even internationally. Competition categories are usually further segmented by 5- or 10-year aliquots.

In this chapter the term *older athlete* is broadened to apply to adults aged 65 years and older, particularly those 75 years and older, who continue to exercise at high intensity and frequency, regardless of competition participation and including activities that are not traditional sports. These older athletes experience, at slower rates, the physical declines seen in most adults over time. Training principles remain the same, yet older adults' physiologic functions and maximal performance do not match those of younger adults. In addition, existing health conditions may require changes to exercise routines. Guidance from health professionals can reduce the risks of injury and encourage continued participation in high levels of exercise into late life.

Aging and Maximal Performance

Longitudinal competition records for older athletes participating in sports provide helpful guides to the maximal possible performances as adults age [2]. For example, elite sprinters show very slow but gradual declines in maximal running speed up to age 80 years, when a more precipitous decline appears. This decline in performance is usually attributed to decreased stride length, muscle power, and other changes, which are partially reversible with targeted training, in some individuals [2]. In endurance sports such as marathon running, which require high aerobic and muscle capacity, performance decreases slowly in elite athletes until about age 75 years. The declines in late life appear to be related to age-related decreases in maximal oxygen uptake, due to decreased maximal cardiac stroke volume and heart rate, and other changes (see Chap. 1, physiologic changes with aging). Depending upon the focus—aerobic, muscle strength or power—training can slow these declines [2]. In contrast, injuries and acquired health conditions can interfere with training and performance.

In some studies, declines in female athlete performances appear to occur at a slightly faster rate than those of males, for unclear reasons [2, 4]. Other studies have not observed these gender differences [5]. Smaller numbers of women participating in competitive sports after age 75 years also prevent firm conclusions.

Training Principles

The training principle of progressive overload, that training stresses should be increased over time as physical function improves, remains the same for older adults. The exercise prescription elements of frequency, intensity, and time are also the same. However, *overtraining* from excessive training intensity or frequency, which can lead to decreased performance at any age, is a larger issue in older adults, who appear to need longer recovery times to avoid overtraining [3, 4]. In response, longer intervals of light after hard training days, with decreased frequency of high intensity training, for example, to twice weekly, are recommended for older adults.

Exercise selection is another key consideration: older adults receive greater benefits from functional movements that mirror their daily activities, including sports and recreational activities. The greatest gains may come from multi-joint exercises that require coordination. However, training exercises should not exceed the individual's ability to perform the exercise in a safe and controlled manner.

Regarding endurance, studies show that when athletes over 60 years reduce their activity to lower levels, their VO_2 max, the maximum amount of oxygen used during intense exercise and a measure of aerobic capacity, drops greatly to that of active but non-athletic older adults [4]. If these individuals exercise regularly at high intensities, VO_2max is relatively maintained [4]. Thus, training intervals that include high intensity are needed to maintain aerobic capacity as athletes age. Benefits can be seen with brief (30–60 s) high intensity interval training that is performed at or above maximal aerobic capacity [4].

For young adults cross-training—engaging in activities other than the competitive sport of interest—is recommended for recovery weeks or recovery after an injury [4]. In contrast, for older adults cross-training appears to be beneficial as an alternative to high intensity training days. Some experts attribute this to potential "micro-injuries" occurring in older adults [4]. For example, an older athlete who takes part in marathon training may benefit from substituting cycling or swimming exercises, with similar duration and intensity, for some running work outs, to reduce the risk of impact-related injuries. An additional benefit is that cross-training can reduce boredom and enhance motivation to continue training. Motivation to exercise often changes as athletes age; the chosen exercise focus will affect performance greatly. However, plasticity continues in late life, such that altering training regimens can improve performance in previously relatively neglected physical functions [2].

Older individuals who change or add activities can continue to see performance improvements [2]. Experts report that, in general, older athletes tend to reduce high level training over time, which may reflect that this level of training is both difficult and less comfortable. Alternatively, the performance expectations for older athletes

Table 11.1 Training considerations for older athletes

Consideration	Rationale	Recommendation
Overtraining	Older adults at greater risk from overtraining	Add more "light" days after a "hard" day, e.g., limit to 2 "hard" days per week Use cross-training after hard workouts, as well as for recovery weeks
Decline in peak endurance	More rapid loss of VO_2 max with lower intensity training Other physiologic age changes	Frequent short bursts (30–60 s) of high intensity training, to maintain high levels of fitness
Loss of muscle mass, power	Physiologic changes with age Older adults may neglect strength training while focusing on endurance	Include resistance/strengthening exercises twice weekly Adequate protein intake
Fall risk	Physiologic changes, including reduced touch, proprioception, and bone density Lack of activities that challenge balance	Include balance exercises most days of the week Evaluate risk for bone loss in men as well as women Adequate calcium intake (women)
Muscle and joint pains	Increased muscle stiffness with age High prevalence of osteoarthritis in older adults Arthritis related to prior injury	Factor impact of exercises into regimen Add stretching exercises most days of the week Pre-treat with analgesics such as acetaminophen and topical non-steroidal anti-inflammatory medications (NSADs); oral NSAIDs may be appropriate for some older adults

have been historically underestimated, which may influence counseling of older athletes by their trainers [2]. Thus, carefully matching exercise modalities to the evolving goals of an older athlete is required (see Table 11.1).

Age-Related Changes

Older adults, even older athletes, experience decreased lean body mass and increased fat over time. Throughout the body, fat distribution changes with an increase in fat deposits in normally lean tissues such as muscle. Such fat infiltration reduces muscle quality (i.e., function relative to size) and can interfere with the muscle's adaptive capacity. In addition, muscle composition characteristically shifts with the portion of Type II fibers decreasing and Type I muscles fibers increasing, and with all muscle fascicles becoming shorter and less angulated [6]. These age-related changes result in a disproportional reduction in muscle function for short duration, high intensity activities such as sprinting, jumping, and reactive movements, in comparison with sustained lower intensity activities such as jogging, swimming, and rowing.

Bone mineral density also decreases in most women after menopause and more gradually in men, with resulting osteopenia, osteoporosis, and risk of fracture with minor trauma such as a fall from standing. Maintaining bone requires exercises with skeletal loading, such as resistance-type training, which many older adults tend to reduce in favor of endurance activities in late life. Older adults focusing on cycling and swimming training should note that these forms of training do not promote bone health as well as walking or running, and have been reported, in younger individuals (e.g., elite swimmers to reduce bone density if performed at high volumes).

Tendon function often changes with age, with resulting changes in the transfer of impact and muscle force to bone in some areas. For example, decreased Achilles tendon stiffness can reduce the rapid transition from the braking to push-off phase in running. It is not clear whether reduced Achilles tendon stiffness is due to aging or to older adults' choices, i.e., to reduce muscle strengthening exercises [2]. Observed decreases in older runners' stride length and ground reaction forces may improve with heavy-resistance exercises, explosive types of weight training, and plyometric exercises [2, 4]. However, because tendons experience reduced regenerative capability with aging, due to biological and compositional tendon changes, it is important to increase recovery time after such activities to reduce the risk of tendinopathy [7].

Balance characteristically declines with age, although it is difficult to separate the effects of aging from co-morbid conditions (e.g., visual changes, osteoarthritis), medications, and reduced participation in activities that challenge balance. Balance is essential to avoiding falls and safely engaging in high levels of most sports and recreational activities [8]. If not already a consistent component of an older adult's regimen, balance exercises must be added. This is particularly important if the target activity does not challenge balance, such as swimming. (See Chap. 4, types of exercises).

Vision is affected by aging, with some changes reversible, such as with corrective lenses and cataract extraction. Other changes, such as decreases in close vision and color discrimination, increased glare, and eye irritation from dry eyes, are less modifiable and may need to be factored into training plans. Vision is essential for avoiding falls and fall-related injuries. and is affected by common age-related eye conditions such as age-related macular degeneration (reducing central vision) and glaucoma (affecting peripheral vision). Studies show that activity levels are lower in individuals with visual loss, yet exercise plays a protective role for many conditions, such as diabetes mellitus, that cause visual loss [9]. With the growth of Paralympic competitions and visually impaired athletes, although visual function must be factored into exercise regimens, it is not a contraindication to continued high levels of exercise.

Tactile acuity, including detection, information relay, and response, commonly declines with aging and affects fine manipulation and performances requiring high touch sensitivity [10, 11]. This is due to intrinsic aging changes as well as extrinsic environmental and lifestyle effects. Peripheral sensation, particularly in the feet, is a key factor in postural stability and maintaining balance [12]. In addition, proprioception, or the awareness of body position in space, can decline with age, medical conditions (e.g., arthritis, diabetes mellitus), and injuries and is critical for strong balance. Examples of proprioception include being able to run without looking directly at your feet or stand on one leg with eyes closed. Joint replacements, particularly knee replacements, remove key proprioception components entirely and exercises such as Tai chi, yoga, and physical therapy are strongly recommended to improve overall proprioception. Over time, older athletes may need to shift away from activities such as ski racing or non-partnered ballet that require excellent proprioception and sensation.

Warm-Ups, Cool-downs, and Stretching

Although high quality research in this area is lacking, cardiologists and sports medicine experts strongly recommend that older adults reliably perform 5 or more minutes of exercises to warm-up before and cool-down after moderate and high intensity exercising [13, 14]. A warm-up should consist of a general warm-up followed by a specific warm-up. A general warm-up includes sustained-low intensity activities, such as walking or cycling, that will gradually increase in intensity over time. The general warm-up gradually dilates blood vessels supplying oxygen to muscles, increases muscle temperature allowing for faster cellular processing, and slowly raises the heart rate, which is thought to minimize stress on the heart. A specific warm-up consists of dynamic stretches with increasing ranges of motion as well as lower intensity movements specific to the activity that will be performed. The specific warm-up provides the same benefits as the general warm-up but also increases flexibility. Stretching is thought to reduce the risk of injury by increasing joint range of motion as well as prepare the older athlete for more intense activities [13]. An example of a warm-up for a tennis player would be 3–5 min walking and light jogging followed by dynamic stretches for the hips, knees, ankles and shoulders, and then practice swings, in a variety of positions, with increasing intensity.

Suddenly stopping intense exercise, while blood vessels to muscles are still dilated from reduced systemic vascular resistance, can cause an older person's blood pressure and pulse to drop [13]. With age, the nervous system may respond less rapidly and effectively to vascular cues. Together these can result in low blood pressure, lightheadedness, and possibly fainting. A cool-down period—slow continuation of the activity—allows a more gradual reduction in heart rate and increased peripheral vascular resistance, with return of blood flow from the periphery. In addition, hydration status is critical for late life athletes as dehydration will promote lower blood pressures. Similarly, ambient heat may affect older adults functioning, including hydration status, more than younger adults. Note that prolonged hypotension after exercising, not related to volume status or anti-hypertensive medications, has been associated with underlying cardiovascular disease and requires evaluation [15].

Stretching after exercise when the muscles are warm is the most effective time to increase flexibility. and can reduce muscle soreness and speed recovery [13]. Most older adults find static stretching after exercise a stress reliever as well. Regular stretching is associated with improved flexibility, range of motion, and posture [16]. Experts strongly recommend regular stretching to prevent or reduce pain related to exercising.

Avoiding Adverse Events

As with younger athletes, keeping to a schedule tailored to the individual, with attention to underlying conditions and past injuries, is essential. After stopping an exercise program, the older adult must resume at a lower level and follow the frequently cited mantra of "start low, go slow." The most common adverse events in older athletes are musculoskeletal complaints, which usually resolve with rest, icing, and elevation. Although experts do not recommend routine cardiovascular testing for older adults engaging in exercise, older adults are more likely to have underlying medical conditions and take medications relevant to training plans [17].

Cardiovascular Events

For older adults and health professionals, usually the greatest exercise-related fear is experiencing a fatal heart attack or stroke provoked by intense activity. Fortunately, research shows that these risks are less for those who exercise than for those who do not [17]. The absolute risk, in numbers, is extremely low: for all age groups, estimates of one sudden cardiac death per 1.5 million episodes of vigorous physical exertion in men and every 36.5 million hours of moderate-to-vigorous exertion in women [18]. Individuals with recent cardiac events, current cardiac conditions, recent strokes, or other cerebrovascular conditions require assessment by the relevant clinician prior to resuming high intensity exercise. Individuals with uncontrolled hypertension, particularly very high readings, similarly require assessment and treatment.

Musculoskeletal Problems

Recovery following an injury in older exercisers often requires more time in comparison to younger persons; pain can persist as long as a year and require adjustments to the exercise regimen [3]. Thus, preventing injury and overuse before an event occurs, through a gradual increase in activity intensity, accompanied by stretching, is recommended.

Research demonstrates that existing joint osteoarthritis and joint replacements are not contraindications to exercise, although they may require changing the level of exercise impact. In fact, exercise is a primary treatment for osteoarthritis (See Chap. 12). Pre-treatment with pain relievers, such as acetaminophen and non-steroidal anti-inflammatory agents (with topical agents preferred over oral agents in late life) is appropriate [3]. For weight-bearing joint replacements in particular, lower impact activities are recommended, which may extend prosthetic life and reduce prosthetic complications [3].

Rehabilitation

After an injury or surgery that pauses exercise routines, rehabilitation is critical for older athletes, to avoid deconditioning with its associated detrimental health effects. Older adults will lose strength and endurance more rapidly than younger persons and inactivity prolongs the return to prior function. Lower impact activities, such as water-based or seated, can be substituted for prior exercise routines during recovery from surgery or significant injury [3].

Summary

Older athletes are proof that the low expectations many health professionals and older adults hold regarding exercise capacity in late life are incorrect. Older individuals who have exercised at a high level for their entire lives usually are able to continue to enjoy high levels of performance into late life, in the absence of certain health conditions. Plasticity continues, such that shifting from a focus on muscle strength to endurance activities, and vice versa, is possible. However, many older adults neglect the critical modalities of muscle strengthening, balance, and stretching, which may need reinforcement by trainers and health professionals. Education regarding increased recovery time and need for warm-ups and cool-downs is essential. Cross-training can be useful for "light" days and for maintaining enjoyment in and motivation for continuing high intensity training. The most common adverse events are musculoskeletal and are treated similarly to those in younger adults, although recovery is likely to be more prolonged with age. Consideration of bone health is important for men as well as women as they age into their eighth and ninth decades.

Case: Part 2

Ann's balance has declined due to loss of proprioception after knee joint replacements: she needs to begin a balance exercise program for most days of the week. After a knee replacement, range of motion can be reduced, thus, continued stretching is important. She might consider snowshoeing or another outdoor activity, instead of cross-country skiing, while improving her balance. Stationary biking is another option. Resistance exercises 2–3 times weekly will be important, to increase and maintain strength. If she lost muscle mass before and after her surgeries, which is common, adequate protein intake and progressive muscle loading are key.

Davis' lightheadedness is likely due to a decrease in blood pressure following intense exercise, with reduced vascular responses with age. He needs to reliably warm-up prior to vigorous activity, such as with dynamic stretches and other low-level activities. He should cool-down, with a slower paced pool length followed by static stretching, after high intensity exercise. Stretching should also help his next day stiffness. As the pool is his only exercise, he needs to add balance exercises most days of the week and resistance exercises 2–3 days weekly. Even if his balance is currently good, it likely will not remain so in the absence of exercises that challenge his balance.

For overall physical function, a balanced program of endurance, resistance, balance, and stretching is most effective and may reduce Ann's and Davis' risk of future injuries, including falls. Given their ages, Ann and Davis should also consult their primary clinician about bone health and fracture risks.

References

1. Lemez S, Baker J. Do elite athletes live longer? A systematic review of mortality and longevity in elite athletes. Sports Med Open. 2015;1(1):16. https://doi.org/10.1186/s40798-015-0024-x.
2. Suominen H. Ageing and maximal physical performance. Eur Rev Aging Phys Act. 2011;8:37–42. https://doi.org/10.1007/s11556-010-0073-6.
3. Tayrose GA, Beutel BG, Cardone DA, Sherman OH. The masters athlete: a review of current exercise and treatment recommendations. Sports Health. 2015;7(3):270–6. https://doi.org/10.1177/1941738114548999.
4. Foster C, Wright G, Battista RA, et al. Training in the aging athlete. Curr Sports Med Rep. 2007;6:200–6. https://doi.org/10.1007/s11932-007-0029-4.
5. Ganse B, Ganse U, Dahl J, Degens H. Linear decrease in athletic performance during the human life span. Front Physiol. 2018;9:1100. https://doi.org/10.3389/fphys.2018.01100.
6. Larsson L, Degens H, Li M, Salviati L, Lee YI, Thompson W, Kirkland JL, Sandri M. Sarcopenia: aging-related loss of muscle mass and function. Physiol Rev. 2019;99(1):427–511. https://doi.org/10.1152/physrev.00061.2017.
7. Lee-Yui PP, Wong CM. Biology of tendon stem cells and tendon in aging. Front Genet Sec Stem Cell Res. 2019;10:01338. https://doi.org/10.3389/fgene.2019.01338.
8. Reimann H, Ramadan R, Fettrow T, Hafer JF, Geyer H, Jeka JJ. Interactions between different age-related factors affecting balance control in walking. Front Sports. 2020;2:94. https://doi.org/10.3389/fspor.2020.00094.
9. Ong SR, Crowston JG, Loprinzi PD, Ramulu PY. Physical activity, visual impairment, and eye disease. Eye. 2018;32(8):1296–303. https://doi.org/10.1038/s41433-018-0081-8. Epub 2018 Apr 3.
10. Correia C, Lopez KJ, Wroblewski KE, Huisingh-Scheetz M, Kern DW, Chen RC, Schumm LP, Dale W, McClintock MK, Pinto JM. Global sensory impairment in older adults in the United States. J Am Geriatr Soc. 2016;64(2):306–13. https://doi.org/10.1111/jgs.13955.

11. Kalisch T, Tegenthoff M, Dinse HR. Improvement of sensorimotor functions in old age by passive sensory stimulation. Clin Interv Aging. 2008;3(4):673–90. https://doi.org/10.2147/cia.s3174.

12. Wickremaratchi MM, Llewelyn JG. Effects of ageing on touch. Postgrad Med J. 2006;82(967):301–4. https://doi.org/10.1136/pgmj.2005.039651.

13. American Heart Association. https://www.heart.org/en/healthy-living/fitness/fitness-basics/warm-up-cool-down. Accessed 8 August 2023.

14. Afonso J, Clemente FM, Nakamura FY, Morouço P, Sarmento H, Inman RA, Ramirez-Campillo R. The effectiveness of post-exercise stretching in short-term and delayed recovery of strength, range of motion and delayed onset muscle soreness: a systematic review and meta-analysis of randomized controlled trials. Front Physiol. 2021;12:677581. https://doi.org/10.3389/fphys.2021.677581.

15. Dubach P, Froelicher VF, Klein J, Oakes D, Grover-McKay M, Friis R. Exercise-induced hypotension in a male population. Criteria, causes, and prognosis. Circulation. 1988;78:1380–7. https://doi.org/10.1161/01.CIR.78.6.1380.

16. La Greca S, Rapali M, Ciaprini G, Russo L, Vinciguerra MG, Di Giminiani R. Acute and chronic effects of supervised flexibility training in older adults: A comparison of two different conditioning programs. Int J Environ Res Public Health. 2022;19(24):16974. https://doi.org/10.3390/ijerph192416974.

17. Gammack JK. Physical activity in older persons. Mo Med. 2017;114(2):105–9.

18. Riebe D, Franklin BA, Thompson PD, Garber CE, Whitfields GP, Magal M, Pescatello LS, American College of Sports Medicine. Updating ACSM's recommendations for exercise preparticipation health screening. Med Sci Sports Exerc. 2015;47(11):2473–9. https://doi.org/10.1249/MSS.0000000000000664.

Chapter 12
Exercise Interventions for Pain Management in Older Adults

Kristi M. King and Jason R. Jaggers

Key Points
- Pain is a multifaceted, acute or chronic clinical condition that increases in prevalence with age
- Pain is strongly associated with poor outcomes for older adults: functional loss, falls, hospitalization, and opioid use disorder
- Research supports that several exercise modalities improve pain from a variety of causes
- Prescreening prior to an exercise prescription should occur to provide adjustments based on the older adult's current health and pain status
- Minor increases in feelings of fatigue or pain should not preclude participation, but dizziness, vomiting, or swollen joints need evaluation prior to continuing exercise
- Activities that include low impact or water aerobics are encouraged
- Long-term goals are to achieve the Centers for Disease Control and Prevention/ American College of Sports Medicine recommendations for exercise for older adults, with modifications as needed

Case: Part 1

Mr. and Mrs. Sampson are 85 years old. She has osteoporosis and exercises most days of the week: zumba, playing tennis, swimming. He describes himself as a life-long "couch potato" who would rather read. She has developed

K. M. King (✉) · J. R. Jaggers
Department of Health and Sport Sciences, University of Louisville, Louisville, KY, USA
e-mail: kristi.king@louisville.edu; jason.jaggers@louisville.edu

© The Author(s), under exclusive license to Springer Nature
Switzerland AG 2024
G. M. Sullivan, A. K. Pomidor (eds.), *Exercise for Aging Adults*,
https://doi.org/10.1007/978-3-031-52928-3_12

moderate right hip pain, which appears due to osteoarthritis, with pain and stiffness especially after exercising. She wants to be able to continue exercising. Mr. Sampson has hypertension, is 40 pounds overweight, and has been told he is pre-diabetic. He takes ibuprofen, a non-steroidal anti-inflammatory medicine, daily for back pain; his physician has asked him to stop this medication, due to his hypertension and kidney risks. He wants to start exercising to help his back pain and prevent diabetes.

Introduction

Currently there are more than 56 million adults ages 65 and older living in the United States (US) or 17% of the population [1]. By 2030 it is projected that the US older adult population will increase to over 20%, or 73.1 million persons [1]. Over half of the US older adult population experiences pain [2] and reports estimate that 80% of individuals living in institutionalized settings, such as nursing homes, experience pain [3]. Pain is a risk factor for problems with physical functioning, independence in activities of daily living, and quality of life [4, 5]. Chronic pain is also one of the most common reasons for adults to seek medical care [6].

It is well-established that engagement in physical activity throughout the lifespan serves to prevent and treat many health conditions, as well as reduce mortality risks [7, 8]. In addition, exercise is an important component for pain management in older adults [9, 10].

Pain in Older Adults

Extensive medical, psychological, and clinical considerations are used in defining pain [11]. In 2020 an international consensus definition describes pain as "an unpleasant sensory and emotional experience associated with, or resembling that associated with, actual or potential tissue damage" [12]. Furthermore, *chronic pain* is pain lasting longer than 3 months beyond the time of typical healing [13] and *high-impact chronic pain* is persistent pain with substantial restriction of life activities lasting 6 months or more [14, 15].

The prevalence of pain increases as individuals age and with the onset of disability [16, 17]. Women and older adults with obesity, musculoskeletal conditions, or depressive symptoms have a higher incidence of pain [2]. Pain is commonly associated with neurodegenerative and musculoskeletal conditions, peripheral vascular disease, and arthritis [5]. The most frequent sites for pain are knees, hips, and low back.

Research indicates that older adults underreport pain and, as a result, may receive inadequate treatment [18]. Studies have also shown that individuals from ethnic and racial minority populations are often under-treated or ignored when reporting pain to healthcare professionals [19–21]. Pain may prevent older adults from engaging in activities of daily living (ADL) [3, 22] and contribute to decreased mobility and falls, poor sleep, cognitive impairment, social isolation, depression, and polypharmacy [23].

Safe, effective pain management is of critical concern: opioid overdose is an increasing cause of preventable accidental deaths [24–28]. Based on current research, opioids are not recommended as a treatment for chronic pain [29] and should be used as a last resort [30, 31]. Older adults, women, individuals with pre-existing conditions, and those from ethnic or racial minority groups, rural areas, or socioeconomically disadvantaged communities are at a greater risk of being inappropriately prescribed opioid prescriptions for pain [32–34].

Exercise Interventions for Pain

Research on exercise interventions demonstrates effectiveness for many types of chronic pain (see Table 12.1). Osteoarthritis joint pain and low back pain are particularly well-studied. These conditions are prevalent in older adults and can cause

Table 12.1 Evidence-based exercise recommendations for pain[a]

Chronic pain type	Exercises	Comments
Low back pain	Lumbar stabilization exercises (balance and elastic band resistance training) Pilates, core strengthening Aerobic Yoga	Yoga poses not recommended for some conditions (e.g., osteoporosis) Back extension may be painful for spinal stenosis Back flexion may be limited in disc disease Use caution in general for flexibility exercises
Knee osteoarthritis	Aerobic Balance Strength Yoga Tai chi Aquatic	Low impact (pool-based, walking, cycling) recommended Start at low intensity
Hip osteoarthritis	Flexibility Aquatic Recumbent cycle Walking	Low impact recommended Stretches can relieve pain
Chronic pain, many causes	Aerobic Strength Flexibility Balance Yoga Pilates Tai chi	Tailor to patient's pain and underlying condition

[a] Initial referral to physical therapy or other specialists is useful in persons with frailty syndrome, falls, low exercise self-efficacy, and other conditions

severe disability. For chronic back pain, guidelines based on moderate quality evidence recommend exercise to improve pain and function [35–37]. In studies, adverse effects from exercise were not serious and were limited to muscle soreness. Among various types of exercise studied—motor control, yoga, Pilates, tai chi—no type has been shown to have a clear advantage; thus, access and personal preference can determine choice [35, 38]. For frail individuals, initiating brief activities with a physical therapist or trainer may be preferable (see Chaps. 1, 6, and 8).

Exercise for osteoarthritis, particularly for knee and hip pain, has been extensively studied. A 2022 systematic review, of 20 studies examining exercise + education vs. education alone for hip and knee osteoarthritis, concluded that pain severity and function improved for exercise + education, without increasing adverse effects [39]. Another systematic review of exercise for hip and knee osteoarthritis found that a variety of exercise types (aquatic, land-based, tai chi, yoga) improved pain, physical function, quality of life, and stiffness, in amounts varying from small to large, without adverse effects [40]. Studies focused specifically on knee pain reveal benefits of exercise for pain [41–43]. A 2022 network metanalysis of 152 randomized controlled trials, of non-steroidal anti-inflammatory medications, paracetamol (acetaminophen), and exercise for hip or knee osteoarthritis, reported that exercise is comparable to these medications for pain relief and function [44]. Based on this substantial work, exercise—aerobic, resistance, and flexibility—is considered first-line treatment for knee and hip osteoarthritis and is recommended in guidelines developed by groups such as the American College of Rheumatology, UK National Institution for Health and Care Excellence (NICE), and American College of Physicians [35, 45, 46].

Studies have also examined the effects of exercise on chronic pain from other causes. A 2017 Cochrane Collaboration systematic review summarized the evidence from 274 studies that examined exercise for multiple conditions: rheumatoid arthritis, osteoarthritis, fibromyalgia, low back pain, intermittent claudication, dysmenorrhea, mechanical neck disorder, spinal cord injury, post-polio syndrome, and patellofemoral pain [47]. Study quality varied and was often low (e.g., small patient numbers with study under-powered to find differences). Types of exercises also varied greatly, in frequency, intensity, and type, with strength, endurance, flexibility, and muscle activation exercises included. Exercise improved physical function and pain severity in small to moderate amounts, in some studies. Adverse events, not aways reported, were limited to increased soreness or muscle pain, of a few weeks duration. Thus, exercise appears to have little downside and potential benefits for chronic pain from many conditions. This finding is in contrast to opinions held by many older adults that exercise for painful conditions will worsen their pain [48].

Implementing Exercise Prescriptions for Pain

Barriers to exercise are even greater for older adults with chronic pain in comparison to other older individuals. Myths about exercise being harmful, even dangerous, for older adults with chronic conditions are pervasive and often held by health professionals as well, despite substantial evidence that exercise is beneficial and risks are low (see Chaps. 2 and 3). Other barriers cited by older adults include time;

access to safe, affordable, or convenient areas; fear of falling and fractures; low self-efficacy for exercise; and lack of motivation [48, 49]. These reported barriers are similar in older adults from various ethnic backgrounds, and in older adults without pain symptoms [50]. Designing exercise prescriptions to respond to these perceived barriers, as well as using motivation interviewing in discussions, will move more older adults with chronic pain toward exercise (see Chap. 5).

Health care and fitness professionals who treat adult patients for pain are ideally suited to recommend safe, effective treatment options for pain while addressing perceived barriers. The American College of Sports Medicine's (ACSM) Exercise is Medicine (EIM)® initiative encourages health professionals to prescribe physical activity when designing treatment plans, and to refer patients to evidence-based exercise programs and qualified exercise professionals [10].

For most older adults embarking on new physical activities at moderate or low levels (e.g., walking), additional evaluations or testing beyond a medical history is not needed, based on decades of research (see Chap. 3). However, in older adults with chronic pain, careful assessment for the most likely cause(s) of pain, pain triggers, and past exercise experience is recommended [7]. For individuals with chronic pain who are frail, or have a falls history or other risks (low vision, cognitive impairment), appropriate consultation to focus the exercise prescription is valuable (see Box 12.1).

Box 12.1 Exercise Training Considerations
General

- Contact and high-risk (e.g., mixed martial arts, boxing, skateboarding, rock climbing) sports are not recommended because of falls and injury risks.
- Low impact activities such as water aerobics or recumbent bicycle are encouraged.
- Because of differences in pain severity and treatment, progression will likely occur at a slower rate.
- Long-term goals are to achieve the ACSM recommendations for aerobic and resistance exercise for older adults, with modifications for symptoms.
- Adjust the exercise prescription based on the individual's age and health status.

Special Considerations

- Supervised exercise, in the community or at home, is recommended for symptomatic (active pain) individuals or those with frailty, falls, and conditions conferring additional risks.
- Individuals should report increases in fatigue or perceived effort, pain, or shortness of breath during activities.
- Minor increases in feelings of fatigue or pain should not preclude participation, but dizziness, swollen joints, or vomiting should be evaluated prior to continuing.
- Individuals with peripheral neuropathy may require adjustment of exercise type, intensity, and range of motion.

When prescribing exercise, it is critical to understand older adults' social and environmental needs and circumstances. Providing information about benefits and safety is helpful to dispel myths, but often not sufficient to respond to other concerns, such as cost or transportation, or to make an exercise program appealing. Does the older adult prefer solitary activities, safe at home? Does the older adult enjoy socializing in a group or being with a few others? If the older adult with chronic pain has not been physically activity, has had negative experiences with physical activity, and/or has low self-efficacy for exercising, a referral to physical therapy or a fitness professional may be the first step forward. Community-based programs are available in many locales, at low cost, and may be an attractive option once an individual has become comfortable with exercising. (See Chap. 11) Unfortunately many communities, especially rural ones, have few resources, including accessible public transportation. Virtual, online programs may fill this gap for some individuals.

Older adults with pain may advance in exercise goals more slowly, but the target remains the same as for all older adults: 30 min daily, 150 min weekly, aerobic and resistance, moderate level exercises, adjusted as needed for each individual [51, 52] (see Chap. 6).

Conclusion

Evidence supports various types of exercise as safe and beneficial for many types of chronic pain in older adults, and more useful than medications. However, older adults are often unaware of these benefits and cite barriers to using exercise as treatment. Additional assessment of the older adult regarding pain causes, and prior treatments and experiences, is useful before initiating an exercise prescription. Health and fitness professionals are ideally suited to prescribe, implement, and lead effective exercise interventions for older adults with chronic pain. In addition, health and fitness professionals can advocate for more universal access to safe, affordable, accessible exercise for all older persons.

Case: Part 2
Initial exercise prescription for Mrs. Sampson's pain:
Mrs. Sampson is referred to physical therapy to learn specific stretches and light exercises to incorporate regularly into her weekly activities. The goal is to reduce pain and minimize the risk of reinjury, while also improving her balance and flexibility, and maintaining her strength. As Mrs. Sampson enjoys swimming, this is a low impact exercise she and Mr. Sampson might do together. Mrs. Sampson also enjoys tennis, but considering her osteoporosis with aggravated hip pain following exercise, she should initially take a step back from the high energy demand tennis places on the body. Another option

for Mrs. and Mr. Sampson may be to play pickleball together a few days a week. Check local organizations or community centers with pickleball for beginners.

Initial exercise prescription for Mr. Sampson's pain:

Mr. Sampson should start by incorporating gentle back and hip stretches most days of the week, since muscle stiffness may be aggravating his back pain. He also needs to begin a slow weight loss program, achieved with gradually increasing his daily activity, without caloric restriction or dieting. Mr. Sampson may be intimidated by his wife's fitness level and the intensity of her recreational exercise activities. Therefore is important to identify activities that both may enjoy. For example, water aerobics is a low impact activity they can do together regardless of differing fitness levels. This activity would help Mr. Sampson increase his activity level gradually and safely, while also reducing risks of pain and injury. In addition, Mr. Sampson should begin balance exercises and low (to start) to moderate (later) intensity levels of resistance training, two days a week. Another option for this self-described "couch potato" which would allow him to watch television, would be exercising on a recumbent bike at a low intensity, for 5–10 min three or more days a week. After a few weeks, if tolerated, he should gradually increase the time by 5 min each week.

Mr. and Mrs. Sampson should be advised to only exercise at a symptom-limited intensity level. They should understand that increasing daily activity may cause some muscle and joint discomfort, but should not be painful. They should stop any activities or exercises that result in aggravated pain, even if delayed.

References

1. Vespa J, Medina L, Armstrong DM. Demographic turning points for the united states: population projections for 2020 to 2060. Washington: U.S. Census Bureau; 2020.
2. Patel KV, Guralnik JM, Dansie EJ, Turk DC. Prevalence and impact of pain among older adults in the United States: findings from the 2011 National Health and Aging Trends Study. Pain. 2013;154(12):2649–57.
3. Cravello L, Di Santo S, Varrassi G, Benincasa D, Marchettini P, de Tommaso M, et al. Chronic pain in the elderly with cognitive decline: a narrative review. Pain and Therapy. 2019;8(1):53–65.
4. Bernard P, Romain A-J, Caudroit J, Chevance G, Carayol M, Gourlan M, et al. Cognitive behavior therapy combined with exercise for adults with chronic diseases: systematic review and meta-analysis. Health Psychology. 2018;37(5):433–50.
5. Dagnino APA, Campos MM. Chronic pain in the elderly: mechanisms and perspectives. Front Hum Neurosci. 2022;16:736688.
6. Schappert SM, Burt CW. Ambulatory care visits to physician offices, hospital outpatient departments, and emergency departments: United States, 2001-02. Vital and health statistics series 13, data from the National Health Survey. Vital Health Stat. 2006;159:1–66.

7. US Department of Health and Human Services, editor. Physical activity guidelines for Americans. 2nd ed. Washington: US Department of Health and Human Services; 2018.
8. US Department of Health and Human Services. Healthy people 2030. 2021. Available from: https://health.gov/healthypeople.
9. King KM, Estill O. Exercise as a treatment for chronic pain. ACSM's Health Fitness J. 2019;23(2):36–40.
10. Medicine ACoS. Exercise is medicine. 2018. Available from http://www.exerciseismedicine.org/.
11. Tesarz J, Eich W. A conceptual framework for "updating the definition of pain". Pain. 2017;158(6):1177–8.
12. Raja SN, Carr DB, Cohen M, Finnerup NB, Flor H, Gibson S, et al. The revised International Association for the study of pain definition of pain: concepts, challenges, and compromises. Pain. 2020;161(9):1976–82.
13. Gatchel RJ, Reuben DB, Dagenais S, Turk DC, Chou R, Hershey AD, et al. Research agenda for the prevention of pain and its impact: report of the Work Group on the prevention of acute and chronic pain of the federal pain research strategy. The Journal of Pain. 2018;19(8):837–51.
14. Von Korff M, Scher AI, Helmick C, Carter-Pokras O, Dodick DW, Goulet J, et al. United States national pain strategy for population research: concepts, definitions, and pilot data. The Journal of Pain. 2016;17(10):1068–80.
15. Dahlhamer J, Lucas J, Zelaya C, Nahin R, Mackey S, DeBar L, et al. Prevalence of chronic pain and high-impact chronic pain among adults – United States, 2016. MMWR. 2018;67(36):1001–6.
16. Molton I, Cook KF, Smith AE, Amtmann D, Chen WH, Jensen MP. Prevalence and impact of pain in adults aging with a physical disability: comparison to a US general population sample. Clin J Pain. 2014;30(4):307–15.
17. Zelaya CE, Dahlhamer JM, Lucas JW, Connor EM. Chronic pain and high-impact chronic pain among U.S. adults, 2019. NCHS Data Brief. 2020;390:1–8.
18. Kang Y, Demiris G. Self-report pain assessment tools for cognitively intact older adults: Integrative review. International Journal of Older People Nursing. 2018;13(2):e12170.
19. Cintron A, Morrison RS. Pain and ethnicity in the United States: a systematic review. Journal of Palliative Medicine. 2006;9(6):1454–73.
20. Goree JH, Jackson J. Do racial and ethnic disparities lead to the undertreatment of pain? Are there solutions? Current Opinion in Anaesthesiology. 2022;35(3):273–7.
21. Hoffman KM, Trawalter S, Axt JR, Oliver MN. Racial bias in pain assessment and treatment recommendations, and false beliefs about biological differences between blacks and whites. Proceedings of the National Academy of Sciences. 2016;113(16):4296–301.
22. AARP, Caregiving NAf. Caregiving in the United States 2020. Washington: AARP; 2020.
23. Gallagher RM, Verma S, Mossey J, Chronic pain. Sources of late-life pain and risk factors for disability. Geriatrics. 2000;55(9):40–4.
24. Rudd RA, Seth P, David F, Scholl L. Increases in drug and opioid-involved overdose deaths - United States, 2010-2015. MMWR Morbidity and Mortality Weekly Report. 2016;65(5051):1445–52.
25. Gostin LO, Hodge JG Jr, Noe SA, Hodge JG Jr. Reframing the opioid epidemic as a national emergency. JAMA. 2017;318(16):1539–40.
26. CDC. Opioid overdose: understanding the epidemic. 2018. Available from: https://www.cdc.gov/drugoverdose/epidemic/index.html.
27. President's Commission on Combating Drug Addiction. President's commission on combating drug addiction and the opioid crisis. Interim report. Washington: President's Commission on Combating Drug Addiction; 2017.
28. Government of Canada. Quick facts on injury and poisoning. 2023.
29. Krebs EE, Gravely A, Nugent S, Jensen AC, DeRonne B, Goldsmith ES, et al. Effect of opioid vs nonopioid medications on pain-related function in patients with chronic back pain or hip or knee osteoarthritis pain: the SPACE randomized clinical trial. JAMA. 2018;319(9):872–82.

30. Schneiderhan J, Clauw D, Schwenk TL. Primary care of patients with chronic pain. JAMA. 2017;317(23):2367–8.
31. Nahin RL. Estimates of pain prevalence and severity in adults: United States, 2012. The Journal of Pain. 2015;16(8):769–80.
32. Dowell D, Haegerich TM, Chou R. CDC guideline for prescribing opioids for chronic pain– United States, 2016. JAMA. 2016;315(15):1624–45.
33. Jones S, Moore L, Moore K, Zagorski M, Brines SJ, Diez Roux AV, et al. Disparities in physical activity resource availability in six US regions. Preventive Medicine. 2015;78:17–22.
34. Weiss AJ, Heslin KC, Barrett ML, Izar R, Bierman AS. Opioid-related inpatient stays and emergency department visits among patients aged 65 years and older, 2010 and 2015: statistical Brief# 244. 2018.
35. Qaseem A, Wilt TJ, McLean RM, Forciea MA, Denberg TD, Barry MJ, et al. Noninvasive treatments for acute, subacute, and chronic low back pain: a clinical practice guideline from the American College of Physicians. Annals of Internal Medicine. 2017;166(7):514–30.
36. Searle A, Spink M, Ho A, Chuter V. Exercise interventions for the treatment of chronic low back pain: a systematic review and meta-analysis of randomised controlled trials. Clinical Rehabilitation. 2015;29(12):1155–67.
37. Demirel A, Oz M, Ozel YA, Cetin H, Ulger O. Stabilization exercise versus yoga exercise in non-specific low back pain: pain, disability, quality of life, performance: a randomized controlled trial. Complementary Therapies in Clinical Practice. 2019;35:102–8.
38. Hayden JA, Ellis J, Ogilvie R, Malmivaara A, van Tulder MW. Exercise therapy for chronic low back pain. Cochrane Database of Systematic Reviews. 2021;9:CD009790.
39. Sasaki R, Honda Y, Oga S, Fukushima T, Tanaka N, Kajiwara Y, et al. Effect of exercise and/or educational interventions on physical activity and pain in patients with hip/knee osteoarthritis: a systematic review with meta-analysis. PloS One. 2022;17(11):e0275591.
40. Zampogna B, Papalia R, Papalia GF, Campi S, Vasta S, Vorini F, et al. The role of physical activity as conservative treatment for hip and knee osteoarthritis in older people: a systematic review and meta-analysis. Journal of Clinical Medicine. 2020;9(4):1167.
41. Dunning J, Butts R, Young I, Mourad F, Galante V, Bliton P, et al. Periosteal electrical dry needling as an adjunct to exercise and manual therapy for knee osteoarthritis: a multicenter randomized clinical trial. Clinical Journal of Pain. 2018;34(12):1149–58.
42. Young JL, Rhon DI, Cleland JA, Snodgrass SJ. The influence of exercise dosing on outcomes in patients with knee disorders: a systematic review. The Journal of Orthopaedic and Sports Physical Therapy. 2018;48(3):146–61.
43. Ettinger WH Jr, Burns R, Messier SP, Applegate W, Rejeski WJ, Morgan T, et al. A randomized trial comparing aerobic exercise and resistance exercise with a health education program in older adults with knee osteoarthritis. The Fitness Arthritis and Seniors Trial (FAST). JAMA. 1997;277(1):25–31.
44. Weng Q, Goh S-L, Wu J, Persson MSM, Wei J, Sarmanova A, et al. Comparative efficacy of exercise therapy and oral non-steroidal anti-inflammatory drugs and paracetamol for knee or hip osteoarthritis: a network meta-analysis of randomised controlled trials. British Journal of Sports Medicine. 2023;57(15):990–6.
45. Excellence NIfHaC. Low back pain and sciatica in over 16s: assessment and management. NICE guideline [NG59]. 2023.
46. Kolasinski SL, Neogi T, Hochberg MC, Oatis C, Guyatt G, Block J, et al. 2019 American College of Rheumatology/Arthritis Foundation guideline for the management of osteoarthritis of the hand, hip, and knee. Arthritis Rheumatology. 2020;72(2):220–33.
47. Geneen LJ, Moore RA, Clarke C, Martin D, Colvin LA, Smith BH. Physical activity and exercise for chronic pain in adults: an overview of cochrane reviews. The. Cochrane Database of Systematic Reviews. 2017;1:CD011279.
48. Lees FD, Clark PG, Nigg CR, Newman P. Barriers to exercise behavior among older adults: a focus-group study. Journal of Aging Physical Activity. 2005;13(1):23–33.

49. Ziebart C, McArthur C, Lee L, Papaioannou A, Laprade J, Cheung AM, et al. "Left to my own devices, I don't know": using theory and patient-reported barriers to move from physical activity recommendations to practice. Osteoporosis International. 2018;29(5):1081–91.
50. Mathews AE, Laditka SB, Laditka JN, Wilcox S, Corwin SJ, Liu R, et al. Older adults' perceived physical activity enablers and barriers: a multicultural perspective. Journal of Aging Physical Activity. 2010;18(2):119–40.
51. Geneen LJ, Moore RA, Clarke C, Martin D, Colvin LA, Smith BH. Physical activity and exercise for chronic pain in adults: an overview of cochrane reviews. Cochrane Database of Systematic Reviews. 2017;4:CD011279.
52. CDC. How much physical activity do older adults need? 2023. Available from: https://www.cdc.gov/physicalactivity/basics/older_adults/index.htm.

Index